How to Succeed After 55

A Roadmap to Success, Good Health, and Happiness

M. M. Amon

Profound Publishers

Copyright © 2023 Amon Mpagazehe

All rights reserved. No part of this publication may be reproduced, stored in a retrieval system, or transmitted, in any form or by any means, electronic, mechanical, recording, or otherwise, without the prior written permission of the author, except in the case of a reviewer, who may quote brief passages in a review to print in a magazine or newspaper, or broadcast on radio or television. In the case of photocopying or other reprographic copying, users must obtain a license from the Canadian Copyright Licensing Agency.

ISBN (Paperback): 978-1-7389199-0-1
ISBN (eBook): 978-1-7389199-1-8

Book design by Aaxel Author Services
Cover design by Matt Swann Creative

Printed in Canada

This book is dedicated to my son, Brian, and his wife, Leila, who stood by me throughout the time I was writing this contribution to the world. It's also dedicated to all my brothers and sisters from all-over who have an open mind, an ambitious heart, and a fiery spirit.

I know that if you have these three things, you have everything you need to design the life and lifestyle you desire. I hope this book can provide a little assistance and inspiration in becoming successful, super-healthy, and maximize all of what your life was meant to be.

DISCLAIMER

This book is for your education and reference. It is neither a medical manual nor a guide to self-treatment for medical problems. The author is not a medical doctor, and neither prescribes treatment nor treats medical problems and does not intend that you attempt to do so either. Use the information here to help you make informed decisions, not as a substitute for any treatment that your doctor may have prescribed for you.

The information and opinions expressed in this book result from careful research. The author believes they are accurate and sound, based on the best judgment available to him. Neither the editors nor the author assumes any responsibility for damages or losses incurred because of using the information in this book, nor for any errors or omissions. It is the responsibility of each reader to exercise good judgment in using any information in this book.

CONTENTS

Introduction 1

My Story 5

CHAPTER ONE: Define Your Own Success 9
    The Guiding Questions to Success 10
    Believe in Yourself 13
    It's Never Too Late 14
    Personal Life Mission Statement 15

CHAPTER TWO: Fundamentals of Achievement .. 17
    Accept Total Responsibility for Your Situation 18
    Avoid Emotional Contagion 19
    Mediocrity Is the Biggest Success Killer 21
    The Compounding Development Effect 23
    Make Excellence Your Priority 25
    Questions to Ask Yourself in Life 27
    Embrace Growth Mindset for Success 30
    Conclusion 32

CHAPTER THREE: How to Fuel Success and Conquer Anything 35
    Simple Moves to Your Next Level 36
    The Hard Truths about Success 37
    Skills You Need to Succeed at Almost Anything 39
    Goals Are Essential to Getting What You Want 42
    Action Is the Key to Success 47
    Move Like and with the Universe 48
    Go Public with What You Want 49
    You Need People to Get Stuff Done 50

Make a Positive Connection 51
　　Keep Up with Rapid Pace of Change .52
　　Mastermind Your Way to Success 53
　　Embrace Persistence 54
　　Maximize Your Personal Energy 55
　　Matching Mental State to Productivity 56
　　Work Harder and Smarter 56
　　Sitting Position 58
　　Tidiness 58
　　Don't Fear, Ask 59
　　Prioritize 60
　　The Joy of Living 60
　　A Word of Wisdom 62

CHAPTER FOUR: Money Mastery 63
　　It's Your Right to Have Money 63
　　Understanding the Rules of Money 64
　　Money Grows When We Spend Less Than We Earn 65
　　Stay Active, Make Money, and Strive in Old Age 67
　　Pay for Every Purchase with Cash 69
　　Eliminate Unnecessary Daily Expenses 70
　　Avoid Being in Debt 70
　　Live Beneath Your Means 71
　　Take Care of What You Have 72
　　Wear Out Everything You Own 72
　　Consider What You Need Before Buying 73
　　Research Your Purchases 74
　　Comparison-Shopping and Bargaining 74
　　Meet Your Needs with Substitutes 75
　　Spending Money Wisely 75
　　Invest a Portion of Your Money Every Month 76
　　Bad Spending Habits to Avoid 77
　　Good Spending Habits to Embrace .79
　　You Better Be Selfish 87
　　Spend Your Money for Maximum Happiness 87

Good Financial Management for Every Older Adult 89
The Financial Situations of Older Adults 90

CHAPTER FIVE: Global and Personal Lifelong Learning 93

What Is Lifelong Learning? 94
Key Differences Between Lifelong Learning and Education. .95
How to Adopt Lifelong Learning? 95
How to Learn the Right Knowledge? .96
Becoming Tech Savvy Is All You Need. 98
Other Important Things You Can Do Because of Lifelong Learning
. 102
Benefits of Lifelong Learning 104

CHAPTER SIX: Embrace Humor for Happiness and Success. 107

Humor Is a Learnable Skill 109
Why Humor Is a Key to Success 109
Humor and Smile Lead to Happiness and Success 114
How to Develop Your Sense of Humor 116

CHAPTER SEVEN: Practicing Gratitude Makes Our Lives Richer 125

The Purpose of Gratitude 126
How to Practice Gratitude. 127
Gratitude Is the Key to Unlocking Happiness and Success. .130
Happiness and Gratitude Increase Goal Success 131
Why Being Grateful Is Important. 131
Conclusion. 136

CHAPTER EIGHT: Happiness Is the Key to Success 139

The Science of Happiness 139
Happiness Leads to Success at Work. 140
Different Definitions of Happiness. 141
Varied Results and Views on the Cause of Happiness. 143

    Happiness Lifts Your Spirits 145
    The Global Pursuit of Happiness 149
    Measures of Happiness 150

CHAPTER NINE: Brain Health Is Central to All Health and Success 153
    You Must Become a Brain Warrior 153
    Memory Is Life 154
    The Memory Rescue Promise 154
    The Brain Is Divided into Four Regions 156
    Blood Flow Is Critical for a Healthy Memory 157
    Blood Flow Risk Factors 158
    Strategies to Support Your Blood Flow 159
    Impact of Toxins on Your Brain and Memory 161
    Strategies to Reduce Your Exposure to Toxins 165

CHAPTER TEN: Happy Aging and Longevity Are the Greatest Wealth 169
    How to Slow Down Secondary Aging? 170
    Habits That May Make You Live Longer 176
    Conclusion 190

Acknowledgments 195

Index 197

Introduction

Writing this book is a dream come true for me. It has always been a dream of mine to find a way to help people, to inspire people, to be of service in some way, and to empower people to be the best that they can be. I truly believe that we all have greatness within us if we just allow ourselves to let go of all our fears, doubts, worries, and all those limitations that are holding us back from achieving our dreams.

What if I told you, you could assure your own success?

What if I told you, you could attract attention and influence people?

That you can have the results you desire?

That you can succeed in any endeavor you want?

That you can achieve your goals—whether they relate to your health, wealth, or happiness?

That you can boost your overall brain power?

That you can supercharge your brain and reverse memory loss?

That you can enhance your likeability?

That you can slow the aging process?

What would you do?

Would you do what it takes?

You're probably thinking, "What's the catch?" Well, there is one, to be precise. I have deliberately put these caveats in this introduction so that if you decide they are unreasonable, you can stop reading now and save your time.

First, you must follow all the advice, recommendations, and strategies that I have laid out in the following chapters. After all, expecting to achieve the results you desire without using the roadmap and tools contained within this book would be bordering on foolishness.

And second, be open-minded when an idea's relevance is not immediately obvious, or if it challenges your existing world view. Do not reject something that is new to you until you have applied it without skepticism for a reasonable amount of time.

This is all I ask.

Humans are more resourceful than we realize. We are the only species on the planet who can create at will. We are the only species who can influence our circumstances. We are the only species who can solve complex problems. Despite this, the vast majority find themselves stuck without choices and confused.

Why is this? There is no simple answer, but my intent for this book is to provide you with solutions so you can step into the person you know in your heart you were meant to be. I know there are many books on motivation, inspiration, and positive psychology already out there, so why read *How to Succeed After 55*?

You're more than a body and a mind, and this book will help you realize your potential. It will enable you to understand your true powers and give you an integrated and holistic approach to unleash these inner powers so you can create the life and lifestyle you truly desire.

I have been a voracious student of success for over five decades. Not just a student who delves into theories, but a practitioner of all I have learned. Dear reader, being a practitioner, I have passion to transfer what I have learned and applied to you.

I have studied many schools of thought, from traditional

psychology, neuroscience, philosophy, and metaphysics, to spirituality and more. Why? Because I found myself on an insatiable journey to figure out why most people struggle to create the life and lifestyles they want.

What I will share in How to Succeed After 55 are time-tested and proven principles, strategies, and tools to enable you to redesign yourself. I will take you through the entire process to help you understand what you need to *know*, what steps you need to *apply*, and how you need to apply them to *guarantee* your success in virtually all areas of your life.

You will learn how to think, how to gain control over your emotions, how to direct your actions, and how to create the results you want. This is what makes this book different from most success-based literature, which are incomplete, because either:

- Do not consider all the internal factors that lead to self-mastery (the most fundamental prerequisite to complete success).

- Do not consider all the external factors that lead to the understanding of the material world.

- Do not teach well-researched laws, principles, and strategies that have their roots in science as well as philosophy.

- Do not teach applied and proven tactics.

- Do not teach the importance of lifelong learning.

My Story

I was born in Rwanda quite a while ago, and a few years after the dust of the Second World War had settled. I do not recall many happy moments from my early childhood, or indeed, much at all from this time, but I do remember my neighbors and relatives being poor and not having peace of mind. Most people around me were illiterate, struggling, and suffering from diseases that are non-existent today.

There was a lot of talk about God and superstition from people around me, but looking back, I realize it came from a place of fear, ignorance, and poverty. I remember not understanding the way in which people talked about certain things or why they behaved as they did. For example, I couldn't understand why many parents didn't care about sending their children to school.

Fortunately, when I was a young boy I went to school, thanks to my parents, who had been educated by the Swiss and American missionaries and knew the importance of education. I remember being excited when praises were lavished upon me by my teachers because I performed well on most exams. I was considered a rising star.

No sooner had I finished high school than I got a British Council scholarship to learn English at the then Makerere University College in the neighboring country Uganda. At the completion of a two-year English language course, I returned home, where I was trained in journalism and radio broadcasting by German expatriates from Deutsche Welle who were in Rwanda under the development cooperation between Germany and Rwanda. All this happened in the early 1960s.

I liked journalism and being a broadcaster, but my long-term goal, backed by a burning desire, was to continue my studies. I finally left my job and enrolled at Long Island University with headquarters in New York State. Its four-year undergraduate program enabled me to study at its campuses in North America, Africa, India, and the United Kingdom.

Upon graduation I returned to Africa and made Kenya's capital, Nairobi, my new home. I worked as a teacher and principal at a high school. A few years later, I joined the hospitality industry, working at travel agencies before joining a four-star hotel as a commission agent, sales representative, and finally as a sales executive for some years. With a burning ambition to become self-employed, I left and started a partnership business in electronics products. The business collapsed because I had not done enough consulting with experienced businesspeople in related businesses, nor had I done enough research. When I went out of business, I did not consider it to be a failure, but a good lesson in decision making.

During my years working in the hospitality industry as a sales executive, and later in my own business, I made money by investing in government bonds. Most bonds in Kenya had fixed coupon rates, which means that the interest rate determined at the bond auction is locked until maturity. Investment return of any amount above Kenya's 100,000 shillings in a ten-year bond with a coupon rate yielded 12 percent per annum.

I decided to immigrate to Canada, where I thought there were more opportunities that could help me succeed, and I was right. Success

My Story

in a free country is simple. Get an education and learn to save and invest wisely. Anyone can do it. You can do it. Upon arrival in my new homeland, I decided to study, despite being in my sixties. I took an interpreter's course at Across Languages, an organization approved by the Ontario government. I became an interpreter in English, French, Kiswahili, and Kinyarwanda. I would still be working today if I hadn't lost my hearing.

As soon as I started working, I decided to invest the little money I had. This time I learned how to make money in the stocks market by picking the best market sectors, industry groups, and subgroups. I came to learn that most leading stocks are usually in leading industries. With the help of financial planners and advisors, I became positive, got prepared, and seriously went all in.

Today, I live a life of purpose, passion, and meaning. I'm mentally at peace, physically fit, and healthy in my golden years. I want to inspire you to do the same, so you too can design a holistically successful life and lifestyle for yourself and your family; a life that will allow you to leave a positive footprint in the world. This book is not a one-size fits-all. I would be surprised if there's anything in it that makes sense to all people. I don't know how much you will learn from an avid reader who has read and continues to read thousands of books without specializing in any topic, but if it arouses your interest and curiosity, it may give you a reason to finish it.

I wish I could give you a sure-fire formula for success, but life doesn't work that way. What I can do is describe a model that you can compare with your current way of doing things. The right answer for you might be a combination of what you're already doing and what you're reading here. You are the best judge of what works for you.

What I promise you is that you are holding a compass that will guide you to the apex of your life. If you follow all that you are about to read, you will be able to open the gates to the highest and best version of you.

Are you ready to live a life of opportunity, abundance, and fulfillment? Are you ready to maximize your potential? Let's go!

CHAPTER ONE

Define Your Own Success

"Define success on your own terms, achieve it by your own rules, and build a life you're proud to live." — Anne Sweeney

Success is much more than riches, power, or fame. Success is simply the feeling of satisfaction and happiness one gets from leading a particular way of life or carrying out a particular activity. This means there is no one universal definition of success. It's only you who can define what "success" looks like to you. Your success vision may include going to the International Space Station, owning a fleet of cruise ships, having 3,000 pair of shoes like the former Philippines first lady, Imelda Marcos, or having a lot of money. Or none of these things may be relevant to you.

Success is often defined as the ability to reach your goals in life, whatever those goals may be. In some ways, a better word for success might be attainment, accomplishment, or progress. It is not necessarily a destination but a journey that helps develop the skills and resources you need to thrive.

Perhaps your definition of success includes a network of influential friends, a loving family, an intimate relationship with your partner, financial security, fame, and power. Creating a philanthropic fund for the underprivileged or completing the home of your dreams. Your success vision may also be having free time to enjoy the life you have crafted and feeling all your dreams are fulfilled.

I, however, do agree with Brian Tracy who said "Virtually all of us have four main goals in common. These are (1) to be fit, be healthy and live a long life; (2) to do work we enjoy and be well paid for it; (3) to be in happy relationships with people we love and respect and who love and respect us in return; and (4) to achieve financial independence so we never have to worry about money again." I hope you also agree with Tracy on the above four common goals for humanity. And finally, there is no "one size fits all" success definition.

The Guiding Questions to Success

What Do You Genuinely Desire?

The number one prerequisite to success is knowing what you want combined with having a burning desire.

Knowing what you want + burning desire

Having a desire is the first step towards achieving success. A desire is much more than a hope and a wish. A burning desire becomes the fuel that keeps us going, even when we are held back by challenges. Think back to a time when you had a burning and sustained desire for something. You'll find that in most cases you ended up achieving what you were after, provided your desire was strong and you sustained that desire for a reasonable time.

Desire is the catalyst for high performance.

When we have a consistent desire, our ability to find solutions is also enhanced. We all possess a keen desire for certain things and a lukewarm desire for other things. Therefore, it is important to aim for things where we have a genuine desire, rather than based on other people's opinions.

Where Are You Now?

Before you can figure out where you need to go and what it will take to get there, you need to figure out exactly where you are right now.

Before you can plan for your success, you need to define your current reality. This helps us understand the gap between where we are and where we want to be. But it also helps us identify areas of personal deficiency that need the most work and attention for us to become successful.

Time for a life diagnosis. Rate yourself on the following key areas in your life, and be completely honest:

- Health and fitness
- Meaningful relationships
- Personal finances
- Peace of mind
- Personal growth

How Do You Get to Where You Want to Be?

Bring forward only the things that will help you succeed in the future, instead of being swept in the past. Everyone has experiences, setbacks, challenges, failures, mistakes, and adversities, but you always have a choice of what you carry ahead with you.

Treat every experience as a resource. Think of all your experiences—good and bad—as a library of resources, available anytime you need the wisdom and accumulated knowledge they hold. Experience is your first and best teacher, a powerful source of information tailored specifically for you. *Think bigger than yourself.* Now and then we all find ourselves at a turning point, a time when life seems to be asking us to choose between staying stuck in the same place and moving out for something new where the destination is yet to be determined. If you venture out, the tests and hardships you meet along the way will boost your courage and help you become more than you ever thought possible.

Find your triggers. We all have triggers, and you're the only one who can defeat yours. The secret to permanently breaking through a trigger is finding something greater—whether it's faith or family or your desire to reach your potential and meet your goals. When you overcome your triggers, you overcome any self-destructive behavior that may be holding you back.

Have faith in baby steps. As you know, you don't have to see the whole staircase to take the first step. Keep taking small steps and watch them begin adding up to big results.

Find your line in the sand. Especially in times of change, you need to know who you are and what's important to you, what you'll tolerate and what you won't, where you can say yes and where you can never compromise. When you do, you can ensure you'll stay on track by steering yourself away from the distraction of misplaced priorities.

Reinvent yourself as needed. Reinvention doesn't mean altering who you are or what you are about to do; it may be as simple as a new method of pursuing the same dream.

Why Do You Want What You Want?

Most of us are curious. The older we become, the more we turn away from the *why* questions and start to focus on the *how*. How do I become wealthy? How do I get out of debt? How do I start my own business?

However, these questions will not provide you with the preliminary ammunition you need for success. In fact, they will discourage you and make you quit before you even get started. The *how* is useless, as well as elusive, without the *why*. The *why* will give you the energy, inspiration, and resourcefulness to source the *how*. When you want to quit, it will be your *why* that provides meaning for your actions, which further creates an intense desire for the success you want.

People who achieve great things are those who are more driven by their *why* than their *how*. Ask yourself these questions:

- Why do I want success?

Chapter One: Define Your Own Success

- Why am I reading *How to Succeed After 55*?
- Why do I want to be more informed?
- Why do I want freedom?
- Why do I want financial security?

You must know what you are fighting for. When life gets tough, when you want to quit, when people disappoint you, you will run out of motivation unless you are clear on your *why*. Your *why* will give you a sense of purpose; it will make you feel inspired, make you persevere, and even make you a better human. It will make you relentless. It will make you mentally tougher. So, have a cause that captures your heart.

In fact, the mind is such a powerful instrument, it can deliver to you literally everything you want. But you must believe that what you want is possible. And belief is a choice. It's simply a thought you choose to think repeatedly until it becomes automatic.

Why does the brain work this way? It's because we spend our whole lives becoming conditioned. Through a lifetime's worth of events, our brain learns what to expect next—whether it eventually happens or not. And because our brain expects something will happen in a certain way, we often achieve exactly what we anticipate.

Therefore, it's important to hold positive expectations in your mind. When you replace your negative expectations with more positive ones—when you begin to believe that what you want is possible—you will focus on accomplishing that possibility until you achieve the desired outcome.

Believe in Yourself

Believing in yourself is a choice. It is an attitude you develop over time. Your responsibility is to take charge of your own self-concept and your beliefs. You must choose to believe that you can do anything you set your mind to—anything at all—because, in fact, you can. It might help you to know that the latest brain research now indicates that with enough positive self-talk and positive visualization combined with the proper training, coaching, and practice, anyone can learn to do almost anything at any age.

If you act as if it is possible, then you will do the things that are necessary to bring about the result. If you believe it is impossible, you will not do what is necessary, and you will not achieve the result.

Finally, you bought *How to Succeed After 55* because of your age bracket, among other obvious reasons. Please rest assured that you can succeed at any age; it's never too late.

It's Never Too Late

Success is something almost everyone wants and spends a lifetime hoping for. Some never find it, while others realize it earlier in life. Toni Morrison is a good example of someone who achieved success later in life. This acclaimed novelist of the Black experience has been celebrated for decades for her books, which include *The Bluest Eye*, *Sula*, *Song of Solomon*, and *Beloved*. Did you know that Toni Morrison did not explode in the public eye until 1993 when she became the first African American woman to win the Nobel Prize for Literature? She was sixty-two.

Joe Biden became the president of the United States when he was seventy-eight-years old, and, as I am writing this book in 2022, is widely expected to run for the second term.

One of the most common excuses people use to avoid the risk of chasing their dreams is "I'm too old. It's too late for me. I didn't start soon enough." Well, it's not true. Consider this: You may not recognize the name, but Tom Allen is Britain's oldest yoga instructor, who still teaches at ninety. He didn't start doing yoga until his mid-fifties but has since been passing on his vast experience with flexibility that defies his age. With what started as a means to keep busy and active after retirement, Tom turned his passion into a lifestyle that inspires all ages.

Here's another "not too late" example. As the United States' oldest female BMX bike racer, Kittie Weston-Knauer has the scars to prove she is one tough athlete. She began by competing in off-road bicycle races in the late 1980s and was often the only woman on the track. Now seventy-two years old, Kittie does not intend to slow down. Her passion for biking started as a dare, and she is now the oldest BMX racer in the country and still wins championships.

Besides your belief that it is not too late to succeed, you should also have your life mission statement. Let me explain why this is crucial in your journey to achieve success.

Personal Life Mission Statement

"The two most important days in your life are the day you were born and the day you find out why."— Mark Twain

What is your mission in life? To answer that, think of the one thing that would make you feel as though your time here on Earth has made a difference. It could be something simple.

Having a personal life mission statement brings focus, clarity, and purpose to your life. For Thomas Edison, it was to create an incandescent light bulb, the phonograph, and the motion picture camera which people needed. For Einstein, it was to solve the mysteries of space and time. Mahatma Gandhi's and Nelson Mandela's life missions were fighting for the freedom of their citizens.

A lot of corporations have a mission statement. Essentially, it is a brief description of *what* they want to accomplish and *why* they want to accomplish it. The mission statement serves as a compass for guiding the company's operations.

Having a life mission statement can be inspirational and motivational. It gives you direction in life, which makes other decisions easier. It helps you decide things like where to live, what type of business you would like to start, and helps you choose the kinds of books and entertainment that feed your soul. Your life mission statement can guide your daily actions, and if something derails you, it can get you back on track.

What exactly is a personal life mission statement? It is a one to two sentence motto that articulates how you define yourself as a person or a team member. It identifies your personal or professional purpose and describes why it is important to you.

Here are examples of personal life mission statements from visionaries:

1. "To serve as a leader, live a balanced life, and apply ethical principles to make a significant difference."

    —Denise Morrison, Former CEO of Campbell Soup Company.

2. "To have fun in my journey through life and learn from my mistakes."

    —Richard Branson, Founder of Virgin Group.

What do successful people do? Well, they know what success they want. They know where they're at. They know why they want that success, and they have a guiding philosophy that resembles the above examples of personal life mission-statements.

CHAPTER TWO

Fundamentals of Achievement

The fundamental of success involves the positive development beyond oneself and is a step-by-step process of improving oneself in every aspect of life. Although the process is difficult and requires patience, it benefits those who want to have a successful and happy life. This requires your consistent and continuous performance, which is likely to benefit your family, finances, relationships, etc.

To achieve something that you have never achieved before, you must become someone who you have never been before. We grow and succeed only when we have mastery over ourselves. Those who excel live a productive life, enjoy healthy relationships, and have internal satisfaction. It manifests in self-defined and self-valued achievement that reflects one's efforts.

The key to unlocking personal achievement is the will to win, the desire to succeed, and the urge to reach one's full potential. Some of the key steps one can take in this regard are believing in yourself, setting high but realistic goals, continuing to learn and grow one's skills, challenging yourself to get out of your comfort zone, and having the best people around and being around the best people.

High achievers follow a systematic approach to their success. There are certain achievement principles you need to understand to lay a strong foundation for life success. These principles are time tested and applied by hundreds and thousands of men and women to achieve a brighter future. The fundamentals in this chapter can take you as far as you dare to dream.

These fundamentals may be simple, but they're effective. Most of today's successful people used them to get where they are in life. Let us now learn how to unlock success by using them.

Accept Total Responsibility for Your Situation

"You must take personal responsibility. You cannot change the circumstances, the Seasons, or the winds, but you can change yourself." —Jim Rohn

One of the most pervasive myths in our culture today is that we are somehow entitled to a great life. That somehow, somewhere, someone— not us—is responsible for our results, circumstances, and success.

There is only one person responsible for the life you're living. You guessed it. This person is you. To become successful, you must embody the perspective of taking 100 percent responsibility for everything you experience in your life. Now, what happens a lot of the time is that we either take partial responsibility, or in many cases, we take no responsibility. But even when you are not directly responsible for something that happens to you, by taking it on, or by acting as though you are 100 percent responsible, you end up empowering and differentiating yourself.

When you take full responsibility for your results, achievements, relationship quality, health and fitness, income and debts, feelings, and actions, you start to feel overwhelmed, because you understand that control over your life lies within you.

This undertaking has two components. The first is taking ownership of your behavior and its consequences. Until responsibility is accepted for your actions and failures, it is difficult to develop self-respect. It is also difficult to gain respect from others. Everyone makes mistakes, poor choices, and fails to act when they should. Even when we do not decide, we make a choice. But you are not the first person, neither will you be the last, to fall short in the behavior department.

The second component of taking 100 percent responsibility is indirect responsibility. This means moving beyond yourself and acting to help in situations around you. This can be calling for assistance in a situation you are not responsible for. In this case, the key is not that you feel you're taking it on but feeling a moral responsibility to help and earn respect and attention. Accepting responsibility, both personally and indirectly, helps define character. When the moment comes to choose responsibility, what you do or don't do tells others who you really are.

If you are serious about having more success in your life, it's time to stop looking outside yourself to explain why you don't have the life and results you want. Ultimately, you create the quality of your life, and you are your results. You. No one else. And to achieve major success in life, to achieve the things that are meaningful to you, you must assume the highest percentage of responsibility for your life. Nothing else will do.

Avoid Emotional Contagion

One of your steps to success is to avoid emotional contagion. Emotional contagion is the ability to influence the emotions and behaviors of others, either directly or indirectly. The etymology of "contagion" is associated with the conscious and unconscious acts of sharing our emotions with others via verbal or physical expression. Though the word "contagion" sounds intimidating, emotional contagion is used as a strategy in work settings and relationships. Our brain adapts to an "emotional culture," and this helps us to read others' emotions to determine how to respond appropriately. Neurologists have found that major neurons are responsible for this phenomenon and are a useful learning tool.

Some people are more sensitive to emotional contagion than others. Because it can influence thoughts and feelings, the results are changes in mood as well. It is important to note that there are certain moods and personalities that are more susceptible to being "contagious" than others.

Research shows that other people's emotions are facilitated by an interconnected network of cells in the brain that makes up the mirror neuron system. This system is a natural response, much like a high-definition camera, that automatically records the details of other people's facial expressions, tones of voice, and body language, and they mirror these details in us. In other words, people who express strong feelings, emotions, and beliefs (positive and negative) can be "contagious."

Some people are habitually addicted to a toxic way of thinking and living. They don't even realize they have a toxic personality or how they negatively affect others. They will tell you why you can't achieve certain things, and why nobody has become successful doing what you're about to do. They live in a problem zone. They focus on the problem, on complaining, and on blaming, rather than looking for a solution. They'll say, "Why bother? It's not going to work." And you'll end up adopting their philosophy and fail to go after what you want with complete confidence and conviction. And even if you still go after it, it would be with doubt and less passion, which is not conducive to success.

For this reason, it's important to identify people who are supportive of us and our journey. People who radiate positive energy, optimism, and encouragement. True, you're going to encounter both positive and negative people in life but you should do all you can to completely avoid the negative ones. However, when we are conscious of the power negative people can yield through their ability to change our heart and mind, and their tendency to crush our self-esteem or dilute our passion, we can put some distance and boundaries in place.

Setting boundaries is easier when that negative person is an acquaintance or someone we don't see on a regular basis, but it can be hard when it's a family member or a friend. In this case, first try to minimize contact with them, even if it's a parent or close relative. Remember, your first responsibility is to your life. Second, try to become conscious of their negative attitude towards life and decide not to emotionally engage with their ideas or thoughts. You should take this seriously because our subconscious mind does not have the ability to reject a command that we hear repeatedly.

Another way to counteract the effects of negative people is to identify people you admire and make a conscious attempt to spend more time with them (if you can). Of course, some people who inspire you aren't around to hang out with. Read their biographies, books, or blog posts. Watch their videos. Doing this will put you in a more positive frame of mind.

Do all that you can to associate yourself with like-minded people, those who want to develop themselves, like you. People with a solution-oriented approach to life, as opposed to a problem-oriented approach. Don't think success is reserved for those born into well-to-do families who have inherited advantages. You can build a life of success by being in the company of people who have achieved what you want to achieve, or who are on their own paths to success. And the more time you spend with them, the more like them you'll become. Be proactive.

Mediocrity Is the Biggest Success Killer

The biggest success killer is identifying with being average and accepting mediocrity as your way of life. Mediocrity is a personal choice. It's a conscious or unconscious choice to be less than you can be. Without understanding the difference between success and mediocrity, we all risk accepting things that are way below our potential and leading a very average life.

What is wrong with mediocrity? Well, mediocrity never stands out. It's just passable, and it does not result in significant changes and improvements in our own or others' lives. If you want to stand out from the over 8 billion people on the planet, you must avoid it like a plague.

We know from research that no one really enjoys crawling through life and living in mediocrity. If you want to test this theory, ask someone who says "I'm satisfied, I'm happy with my current income or my current situation" one question. Ask them, "If someone offered you a mortgage-free beach cottage worth one million dollars, would you accept it?" You will find most people will say yes if they are being honest.

So, if they want it, why have they settled for less? Well, they have a deep belief that they cannot have more, so they've settled for the ordinary and average. One of the symptoms of mediocrity-based thinking is playing the games of life, or financial freedom, just enough to not lose the game. Most people settle for less than their true potential.

People who accept mediocrity and being average or ordinary often say things like, "It's not good to obsess," and "Life is all about balance." Now you are probably wondering what is wrong with balance. Isn't balance a good thing? Yes, of course it is, but when we balance the objective, we often do it at the expense of diluting energy towards a cause or desirable outcome.

People have been told that it's okay to settle for less, rather than being obsessed with their dreams, because obsession is seen to be a bad thing. When you are obsessed with a good cause, when you're passionate about your craft, and when you don't want to settle for anything less than being successful, you may be seen by others as abnormal, greedy, obsessive, self-serving, or even someone who has never been satisfied, so some of the advice you may get from mediocre people might include:

- Be grateful, someone else is worse off than you.
- Bigger isn't better.

- Don't work too much, too hard.
- Life is short.
- Money or success isn't everything.
- Slow down. Life is to be enjoyed.
- Take it easy.
- It's too late.

What's interesting is that most people who say these sorts of things are obsessed with comfort, with being normal, unmotivated, or purposeless, or with sticking to doubts that prevent them from playing big.

Mediocrity is a formula that works for no one, no matter how much you try to make sense of it. Unhappy people can't teach you how to be happy. Poor people can't teach you how to become wealthy and famous. Look at Martin Luther King, Mahatma Gandhi, Bill Gates, and Jeff Bezos. They did not become superheroes because of their talents—they became great achievers because of their obsessions and unshakable dedication. They didn't just play the game; they were obsessed with winning.

In the next section, we are going to learn about the compounding development effect and how small actions can lead to incredible results.

The Compounding Development Effect

The compounding development effect is a very powerful success concept, one of the most legitimate I have come across. Everywhere you look these days, people are offering quick solutions, tips, and tactics in blogs and articles about how to become more successful, wealthy, sexy, or how to lose weight. Realistically, there is no quick fix when it comes to sustainable success. Of course, it's possible for people to lose weight or make money quickly; however, it's not possible for people to sustain that instant level of success, wealth, or their ideal weight without understanding the compounding development effect.

The compounding development effect, also called the compounding effect, is based on the most time-tested fundamental principles of success. The formula is this:

Small, Smart Choice + Consistency + Time = RADICAL DIFFERENCE

The compounding effect is the principle of reaping huge rewards from a series of small, seemingly insignificant but smart choices. This strategy works in any area, whether you're trying to improve your finances or anything else, it doesn't really matter. If you're standing in front of an audience and ask: "If you had the choice between a million dollars today or having one cent that simply doubles for the next thirty-one days, which option would you pick, and why?" Of course, most people will know it's a trick question. But here is the thing: most people, if confronted with the choices, would probably succumb to instant gratification and take the million dollars.

Very few people, if any, would opt for the one-cent option. And yet if they did take the one-cent option and allowed that money to double every day for the next thirty-one days, that one cent would be worth 10.7 million on the thirty-first day. *This is because of the power of compounding interest.*

For someone who doesn't understand the compounding effect and its applications, it is very probable that they would regret their decision, even if they did opt for the one-cent option. Do you know why? Because, if they did go for that option, even on the twenty-sixth day that money would be worth only $336,000, and they wouldn't realize that in the final five days that would leap to 10.7 million. From the first day to twenty-sixth, the money grows in very small increments. This is one reason most people do not become wealthy—they do not understand the compounding effect.

So, the compounding development effect works this way: If you're improving yourself in small, smart ways over time, you may not see much change for a while. But there will come a day you see massive improvements and results in your life. It works in reverse as well. If you neglect things that you should not be neglecting, you may not see negative repercussions in the short term, but in the long-term things will go from bad to worse. It's like a crack in a windshield. You can prevent the glass from shattering if you get it fixed quickly, but if you allow the crack to go unattended for a long period of time, it may grow larger and larger, or shatter the glass.

The compounding effect is the only process a person needs to achieve the ultimate level of success. People should not be tempted by the promise of quick success, because the path to success can be laborious, tedious, and sometimes a very boring endeavor, but having wealth, influence, and becoming world-class is possible for anyone if they follow through on what needs to be done.

In the following section we are going to learn how making excellence your priority can be a powerful tool for success.

Make Excellence Your Priority

We as humans always dream of fame, success, and growth. We struggle to live to our highest potential and to achieve growth and excellence on a personal, professional, and academic level. Many of us are aware of what it takes to grow and succeed, but most of us don't know how one can be successful and can achieve excellence on all levels. We must make excellence our top priority in all aspects of our lives, and it can be achieved by always striving to do better.

Excellence is the condition of surpassing our standards of expectations. Many people around us who do not strive for excellence have a hard time and do not feel happy with their lives, while people who always strive to achieve excellence feel happy, have inner satisfaction, and contribute positively to others as well. Personal excellence is a lifelong process of developing mental and emotional skills to do better in all aspects of our lives.

The following are examples of steps that can help you achieve personal excellence.

1. Personal SWOT

SWOT is a strategic planning and management technique used to help a person or organization identify *strengths*, *weaknesses*, *opportunities*, and *threats* related to business competition or project planning. Knowing your strengths, weaknesses, thoughts, and emotions, as well as life principles and beliefs, is the foundation in gaining personal excellence as it helps you understand yourself deeper, explore your mind, thoughts, and attitudes, and understand how you deal with challenges. In this step you should think critically about your thought processes and emotions and understand your core beliefs and identify your life principles.

2. Identifying Key Skills Sets

We all have different skill sets and they vary from individual to individual. In this step you should identify your skill set. When identified, you utilize them to make yourself better and better in the process.

3. Know What You Love

You are satisfied and happiest when you are doing things that you love the most, and you enjoy well. Thus, knowing what you really love to do is key to gaining personal excellence. You should evaluate yourself, understand yourself and what you are good at, and what you love to do in all aspects of life.

4. Identify Your Life Goals

Once you know your strengths, weaknesses, skill set, and what you love, the next important thing is to identify and define your life goals. Once you do, your journey to achieving all that your heart is burning for will be tremendously easy.

5. Make an Action Plan

A detailed action plan makes personal excellence achievable. It's critical that you make one once you go through the above steps. Define step-by-step actions that you will take to achieve your personal excellence—making you the best version of yourself.

6. Revisit and Strategize Yourself

You should follow the same steps again and again to explore yourself more, revisiting your action plan and strategizing it, to make yourself perform greater and greater. This is how you gain personal excellence, when you are continuously working to improve yourself.

Questions to Ask Yourself in Life

Believe it or not, these kinds of questions affect the life you lead. That's because the questions you ask yourself literally determine what your mind focuses on, triggering certain thoughts, actions, and inactions, ultimately affecting the results you see in life.

To the extent you focus on self-limiting, negative questions, you will get self-limiting, negative answers and the same unhappy reality. However, when you shift to ask yourself empowering, deeply reflective questions, your consciousness shifts to a whole new level and sets into motion the thinking and actions required to jumpstart your life.

I believe questions are a key to self-awareness and personal growth, and this section contains vital keys to unlock important answers within you. If you've never asked yourself these questions before, it's normal for your mind to draw a blank. That's okay. Simply spend some time thinking over each question and let your mind run free. Ask them over and over, at different sittings. Soon the answers will come to you.

Also, know that there is no one final answer. Your answers today may be different one, two, three years from now, and that's part of your personal growth journey. You may want to use a journal to record your answers, then refer to them years down the road to see how you've changed and grown.

I present to you, many questions to ask yourself:

1. Who are you?
2. How would you describe yourself?
3. What are you passionate about?
4. What personal achievements are you most proud of?
5. What are you most grateful for?
6. What are the most important things to you in life?
7. What are your values? What do you represent? What do you want to embody?
8. Do you love yourself?
9. Why or why not? What do you love most about yourself?
10. How can you love yourself more today? What is your ideal self?
11. Look at your life now. Are you living the life of your dreams? Why or why not?
12. If you had one year left to live, what would you do?
13. If you had one week left to live, what would you do?
14. If you had one day left to live, what would you do?
15. If you had one minute left to live, what would you do?
16. What would you do today if there were no tomorrow?
17. What are the biggest things you've learned in life to date?
18. Is there something you're still holding on to? Is it time to let it go?
19. What are you busy with today? Will this matter in one year? Three years?
20. What opportunities are you looking for now?

Chapter Two: Fundamentals of Achievement

21. How can you create these opportunities?
22. What are your biggest goals and dreams?
23. Is there anything stopping you from pursuing them? Why? How can you address these factors?
24. If you were to do something for free for the rest of your life, what would you want to do?
25. What would you do if you could not fail; if there were no limitations in money, resources, time, or networks?
26. What do you want to achieve in one year? Ten years?
27. What is your ideal life?
28. What can you do to start living your ideal life?
29. What do you fear most in life? Why?
30. What limiting beliefs are you holding on to?
31. What empowering beliefs can you take on to help you achieve your goals?
32. What bad habits do you want to break?
33. What good habits do you want to cultivate?
34. What are the biggest actions you can take now to create the biggest results in your life?
35. Are you living your life to the fullest right now?
36. What is the meaning of life?
37. What is your life's purpose? Why do you exist? What is your mission?
38. How can you make your life more meaningful, starting today?

39. What drives you?
40. What are the times you are most inspired, most motivated, most charged up?
41. Who are the five people you spend the most time with?
42. Are these people enabling you or holding you back?
43. Who inspires you the most?
44. How can you be like them?
45. Are you afraid of letting others get closer to you? Why?
46. Who is the most important person to you in the world?
47. Are you giving him or her the attention you want to give them?
48. How can you spend more time with them starting today?
49. What kind of person do you enjoy spending time with?
50. Who do you want to be like in one year? Three years? Ten years?
51. Who are your mentors in life?
52. What is one thing you're going to do differently after reading all these questions?

Let us now move on to the next section to learn about *growth mindset*, an important attitude which determines how an individual will interpret and respond to a situation. It plays a crucial role in personal development.

Embrace Growth Mindset for Success

The concept of mindset was first discovered by world-renowned Stanford University psychologist Carol Dweck. A mindset refers to whether you believe your intelligence is fixed or changeable. But how do we have different mindsets? Our mindset is formed and developed in our childhood years by our parents, teachers, and friends. We absorb what we see, hear, and experience, and as we have little or no point of reference at this time, we reinforce this knowledge, which becomes deeply embedded in our subconscious mind. With that we then believe about how the world operates and our place in it, and that is how our fixed or growth mindset is formed.

Having a *growth mindset* means you understand that you can improve or learn more if you put in the effort. On the contrary, people with a *fixed mindset* may say they're not a "math person" to avoid practicing math. While they can prevent momentary failure and struggle with this excuse, they are putting off the opportunity to learn, grow, and develop new skills. A person with a growth mindset would be willing to attempt practicing math, even if they struggle and fail during their first try. People with a growth mindset view failures and setbacks as an opportunity to grow and as a sign that they should continue to develop their skills.

Your mindset plays a critical role in your success and how you cope with life's challenges. Those with a growth mindset show greater resilience and a burning desire to learn and succeed. They see failure as feedback, challenges, and an opportunity to learn and grow.

I'm going to give you an opportunity to see whether you may have some of the fixed mindset traits in yourself. Here they are:

Failure Is the Limit of My Abilities

If you believe this, you have a typical fixed mindset. And yes, you will fail repeatedly! It's how you view your failures that matter though. Thomas Edison failed repeatedly in his attempt to create the light bulb. Those failures finally led him to success, and now we have light in our homes! So, every time we fail it's an opportunity to look at the situation in a whole new light and consider how we could do things differently to create the success we want.

My Abilities Are Unchanging

This statement views our intelligence as fixed and unchangeable. Research, however, shows the brain is much like a muscle in that it needs exercise to stay functional and perform at its best. The idea that intelligence is fixed has become somewhat of an outdated notion.

If we continue to find ways to improve and enhance what we know and can do, then we are providing ourselves with better opportunities and can dramatically shift our results. This is a key approach for any business owner if they want to grow and evolve their business.

Growth mindset has never been more important than now. The world is changing at an incredibly fast pace, and there are new challenges we must face every day. Our way of life is changing, norms are changing, and we must keep up. Therefore, having a growth mindset is imperative.

Conclusion

Discover yourself. Knowing who you are from the inside out is one of the most important parts of having a successful life. You are more than your name, occupation, religion, cultural beliefs, or your educational background. In most cases, people have not picked these things for themselves. They have been inherited through cultural, media, religious, and educational conditioning.

Who you really are should be defined by something deeper: your purpose, passion, vision, values, strengths, and your goals. Unless you know exactly who you are, your decisions will always be based on what your family and friends say, as well as the media's influence.

Your purpose is your compass on your life's journey. Once you understand your purpose, you can dedicate your life to doing what you love to do. You will know what you're good at and will set goals and directions for your life consistent with your purpose. The following are important parts of the compass on your life's journey:

Knowing our values. Our propensity to make bad decisions is significantly reduced when we understand what is important to us—or what our values are. Knowing your values is essential for discovering your purpose and revealing your destiny.

Understanding your strengths. When people want to become more successful, they typically try to identify and correct their weaknesses. When you do, you can leverage your strengths to create the life you want.

Exploring your passion. I cannot express enough the importance of understanding your underlying passion. If you can align your career path, calling, or vocation with passion, you can increase your success in quantum leaps.

I have already covered the importance of purpose, but it is only the initial ingredient of success. Purpose by itself is not sufficient to bring you what you want in terms of success and fulfillment. You also need passion. Passion along with purpose is a formidable combination.

Live the life you want to live. Everyone is searching for success and meaning in their lives. You are not alone in your journey. Your ability to create, achieve, love, strive, risk, and dare is what drives your success. They say you get wiser as you get older. I don't want you to wait because you're already old. Start making these changes today. Start flipping these switches of success.

CHAPTER THREE

How to Fuel Success and Conquer Anything

"Life is like a combination lock; your job is to find the right numbers, in the right order, so you can have anything you want." —Brian Tracy

No matter who you are, where you come from, what you do for a living, or how much money you have, everyone has a shot at success, greatness, and an extraordinary life. It all starts when we feel excited about our lives. We feel young, confident, and alive. Everything clicks. We feel like we are going somewhere, like we have momentum. We become more powerful versions of ourselves.

The powerful you have always been here waiting, like a switch inside you that needs to be turned on! It's the part of you that loves discovery, curiosity, challenges, exercise, connecting with other people, checking off goals, acting, heading somewhere, and talking out loud. It's a force inside you that wants to grow, move, and expand. All you must do is locate the switch and turn it on. Once it's on, work at it constantly, not leaving a stone unturned, and never deferring for a single hour that which can be done now.

This old proverb is full of truth and meaning: "Whatever is worth doing at all, is worth doing well." Often a man acquires a fortune by doing his business thoroughly, while his neighbor remains poor for life because he only half-does it. Ambition and energy, industry, and perseverance are indispensable requisites for success in business and life.

Fortune always favors the brave, and never helps a person who does not help himself or herself. Never hope and wait for something to turn up. Idleness breeds bad habits, and clothes a man in rags.

Most successful people today started out in life poor, with determination, industry, perseverance, economy, and good habits. They went on bit-by-bit making their own money and saving it, and this is the best way to acquire a fortune.

Simple Moves to Your Next Level

When you're at a point where you feel ready to take yourself to the next level, how do you make it happen? When you want to succeed in new ways, what are the next steps you must take? Here are significant ways you can move to the next level:

Grab Your Map and Compass

Even setting out in the spirit of adventure, you need a map so you know where you are, and a compass, so you know what direction you're moving in. Structure your plans so you have both elements firmly in place before you take the next step.

Failure Doesn't Mean the Game Is Over

Learn to be okay with failure, secure in your commitment, and know you won't quit when things get hard. Failure doesn't mean the game is over, it means try again—but this time with experience. Failure is part of life, so don't let temporary setbacks keep you from success. Persistence is the key, so simply refuse to give up.

Chapter Three : How to Fuel Success and Conquer Anything

Reinvent Yourself as Needed

To reinvent yourself means to change how you see the world, your inner programming and self-image. This can take some time and effort, as we often become a certain way because of who we "think" we are and how we see ourselves.

The Hard Truths about Success

Most people desire success, but very few want it badly. Many important aspects differentiate the successful people from unsuccessful ones, which have been discussed in chapter two.

Now everyone sees success as the ultimate happiness and fulfillment. Why? Because celebrities, successful men and women, are always looking good and happy in front of the screen. This has created a general belief that they are. Success doesn't always bring happiness. For each person, and according to each circumstance, success may result in different outcomes. Some of them are good, while some of them are bad. Like with any situation, we must assess whether our expectations of success will bring more benefits than disadvantages.

In most of these cases, success will be worth it, but we must not be ignorant of some truths.

You'll Lose Some Friends in the Meantime

Losing friends in the process is inevitable. Because success is not easy to obtain, you'll have to do more every day. More work means fewer distractions, fewer people in your life, and so on. This cuts a lot of social time because you just won't be able to fit it in. Of course, if you choose to adopt a more flexible lifestyle and set longer-term goals, maintaining a life-work balance will be easier. If you are 100 percent dedicated, you'll cut your circle of friends in half.

You Will Have to Sacrifice Things

Aside from friends, you will have to sacrifice other things too. Your free time, for instance, the time in which you relax, will often be cut off. Sometimes you will have to pull out a seventy-hour week to accomplish your goals because the bigger purpose matters more than free time for now.

Besides the number of relationships that may reduce in time, you'll have to sacrifice certain feelings. For example, being a part of a dedicated, loving relationship takes a lot of energy and time. You can't expect to grow a multi-million-dollar business while spending four hours a day with your partner.

Lots of Tough Decisions

In your journey to success, you'll have to make a lot of decisions. Some of them might turn out to be irrelevant, while some might be critical. Many successful people have ended up broke because of one decision. Just one and you're done.

Being successful often puts the responsibility of making difficult decisions on your shoulders, and when this factor kicks in, life can become even more stressful. Unfortunately, you'll have to deal with it and find ways to adapt.

Everything Is on You

Absolutely correct. Everything falls on you, and you cannot avoid responsibility. Success often means tough choices, challenges, and sacrifices. There is no parent, no boss, no one. You are on your own, and you must make it work.

When problems arise, you must find the solutions on your own, and you'll have to assume responsibility for everything. In chapter two, you learned that you must take 100 percent responsibility for your situation.

You Must Be Adaptable and Flexible

If you truly want to succeed, and even when or if you do, you must be extremely flexible. Life never turns out exactly how we imagine. Things spin out of control sometimes, and we must find a way through.

If you work hard and happen to be successful, figure out whether your version of success is really going to make you feel fulfilled. If it doesn't bring a positive feeling, stop doing it immediately.

Skills You Need to Succeed at Almost Anything

What does it take to succeed? A positive attitude? Well, sure, but that's hardly enough. The law of attraction? These ideas might act as spurs to action, but without the action itself, they don't do much.

Below is a list of skills that will help anyone get ahead in practically any field, from running a company to running a gardening club. Of course, there are skills specific to each field as well, but my concern here is the skills that translate across disciplines, the ones that can be learned by anyone who feels young at heart.

1. Public Speaking

The ability to speak clearly, persuasively, and forcefully in front of an audience—whether of one or thousands—is one of the most important skills anyone can develop. People who are effective speakers come across as more comfortable with themselves, more confident, and are more attractive to be around. Being able to speak effectively means you can sell anything—products, of course, but also ideas, ideologies, worldviews. And you can sell yourself, which means more opportunities for professional advancement, bigger clients, or business funding.

2. Writing

Writing well offers many of the same advantages as speaking well. For example, good writers are better at selling products, ideas, and themselves than poor writers. Learning to write well involves not just a mastery of grammar, but the development of the ability to organize one's thoughts coherently and target them to an audience in the most effective way possible. Given the huge amount of text generated by almost every transaction—from court briefs and legislation running into the thousands of pages, to those foot-long receipts you get when you buy gum these days—a person who is a master of the written words can expect doors to open in just about every field.

3. Self-Management

If success depends on effective action, effective action depends on the ability to focus your attention where and when it is needed most. Strong organizational skills, effective productivity habits, and a solid sense of discipline are needed to keep yourself on track.

4. Networking

Networking is not only for finding jobs or clients. In an economy dominated by ideas and innovation, networking creates the channel through which ideas are created. A large network, carefully cultivated, ties one into not just a body of people but a body of relationships, and those relationships are more than just the sum of their parts. The interactions those relationships make possible give rise to innovation and creativity and provide the support to nurture new ideas until they can be realized.

5. Critical Thinking

We are exposed to hundreds, if not thousands of times more daily information than our ancestors were. Being able to evaluate that information, sort the potentially valuable from the trivial, analyze its relevance and meaning, and relate it to other information, is crucial and woefully undertaught. Good critical thinking skills immediately distinguish you from the masses.

6. Decision Making

The bridge that leads from analysis to action is effective decision making—knowing what to do based on the information available. While not being critical can be dangerous, so too can over-analyzing, or waiting for more information before deciding. Being able to take in the scene and respond quickly and effectively is what separates the doers from the wannabes.

7. Math

You don't have to be able to integrate polynomials to be successful—the ability to quickly work with figures in your head, to make rough estimates, and to understand things like compound interest and basic statistics gives you a big lead on most people. All these skills will help you to analyze data more effectively, and more quickly, and to make decisions based on it.

8. Research

Nobody can be expected to know everything, or even a tiny fraction of everything. Even within your field, chances are there's far more that you don't know than you do know. You don't have to have all the answers, but you should be able to quickly and painlessly find out what you need to know. That means learning to use the Internet effectively, to use a library, to read productively, and how to leverage your network of contacts—and what kinds of research methods are going to work best in any given situation.

9. Relaxation

Stress will not only kill you, but also it leads to poor decision making, and poor socialization. So, by failing to relax, you knock out at least three of the skills in this list. Plus, working yourself to death to keep up, and not having any time to enjoy the fruits of your labor, isn't really "success." It's obsession. Being able to face even the most pressing crises with your wits about you and in the most productive way is possibly one of the most important things on this list.

10. Basic Accounting

It is a simple fact in our society that money is necessary. Even the simple pleasures in life, like hugging your child, ultimately require money, or you are not going to be around to hug them for very long. Knowing how to track your income and expenses is important just to survive, let alone to thrive. More than that, the principles of accounting apply more widely to things like tracking the time you spend on a project or determining whether the value of an action outweighs the costs in money, time, and effort. It's a shame that basic accounting isn't part of the core K-12 curriculum.

What else? Surely there are more important skills that I'm not thinking of now. That's why people like Jeff Bezos, Bill Gates, Elon Musk, and Warren Buffett are likely to know more than what I've just detailed above. Let us now move on to the importance of knowing what you want in life.

Goals Are Essential to Getting What You Want

Some years ago, Yale University researchers conducted an intensive study where they interviewed the graduating class just before they left school. They asked the students a series of questions about how to get what you want, one being: "Do you have a clear, specific set of goals with a written plan for achievement?" Less than 3 percent of the students answered yes. Then, twenty years later, the researchers went back and interviewed the class members again to find out what their lives were like. They noted that the 3 percent who had written out their goals for a specific plan seemed to be happier and more well-adjusted than the others. Of course, that is subjective. But they also found that the 3 percent group was worth more in financial terms than the other 97 percent who did not have clear goals.

The study demonstrates the power of goal setting. Goals allow us to plan for our future in advance and enable us to get what we want. They help us to envision our destinies and shape our lives. They give us direction and hope. But they must be the right goals. Meaningful goals create emotion and drive inside you. They spur you to grow and expand. Not only do they spark a sense of hunger in you, but they allow the other areas of your life to thrive as you pursue your vision. But if you want meaningful goals, then you must create goals that are compelling enough to draw these emotions out of you.

More than that, this goal-setting process goes far beyond merely having a vision for something greater. You need to build the foundation that will give you the skills you need and allow you to pursue your goals without fear. When this foundation is already built, here's what must do next:

1. Fulfill Your Essential Needs

What does it mean to fulfill your essential needs? It all goes back to the six human needs:

- Certainty
- Significance
- Variety
- Love/connection
- Growth
- Contribution

These are the deepest needs of all humans, and they drive everything we do. When these essential needs aren't fulfilled, we get stuck in harmful cycles, unhealthy relationships, destructive habits, addictions, unfulfilled professions, and lives filled with fear instead of joy.

To break these cycles and achieve what you want in life, you must fulfill your essential needs first. Surround yourself with good people. Build authentic relationships. Discover your values and create goals aligned with your truest self. When you're striving, pursuing what you want, you're enriching your life and the lives of others.

2. Overcome Your Limiting Beliefs

Now that you've fulfilled your essential needs, you can focus on your limiting beliefs. These are the stories you tell yourself about the way you are and the way the world is. Such beliefs are often formed in childhood, based on how we were taught to earn the love we desired most, or if our needs went entirely unfulfilled. These beliefs are deeply engrained, but that doesn't make them true. You can change your story, and when you do, you'll change your life. Once you've identified these beliefs, you can be on the lookout for the negative self-talk that creeps into your inner monologue. Replace these negative thoughts with empowering ones that help you get what you want instead of holding you back.

3. Adopt Empowering Habits

Ultimately, a healthy mindset is the basis for getting what you want in life. If you let your emotions and circumstances outside your control dictate your mindset, you'll always be distracted from your end goals. But when you learn how to control your mindset, you can control your outcomes. One way to do this is to adopt empowering habits.

You should embrace meditation because it calms the mind, and when your mind is calm and centered, you're in touch with your true desires, so you're able to make actionable plans to get there. If you are new to mindfulness meditation, you can start a practice in just a few minutes a day.

Gratitude is another habit that can completely transform your mindset. When you realize that life happens for you, not to you, you're able to approach challenges as opportunities instead of obstacles. You'll create a deep belief in yourself and become truly unstoppable.

4. Write Your Goals Down

Write your goals down, not on a computer but in a journal or a physical piece of paper. There is something that happens when we write something down. You become a creator when you write down your goals. You are acknowledging both to your conscious and subconscious minds that where you are now is not where you want to be. Your brain then makes this distinction and becomes unhappy with the status quo.

One of the strongest incentives is a sense of discontentment. When you're totally comfortable and relaxed, you're not going to be inspired to do whatever it takes to make things happen. Discontentment is a power that you want on your side. There is a real drive when you find something that you want to move away from, and tension and pressure can serve as powerful drivers of our actions. Use this as a tool to influence yourself as you start taking actionable steps towards your success. Learning how to get what you want becomes a strategy instead of just a dream.

5. Get Clear on the Why

Have you ever thought about what your goal in life is? Some people live their entire existence trying to answer this question. Some people will find the answer, some will not, and others are sleepwalkers; they don't feel the need for a purpose guiding their actions.

Now, get crystal clear. Write out the details of how achieving your goal would make you feel. What would it mean to you to get what you want? How would it change your life? When you're clear on why your desires are important to you, learning to get what you want (or how to get people to do what you want) becomes more natural.

By getting clarity on why you must achieve your goal, you will find your purpose. And purpose is stronger than outcome. Learning how to get what you want becomes a source of fulfillment, since you're acting in alignment with your passions.

Knowing this purpose will help get you through the rough times and create a strong enough *why* to keep you going. You will have the fuel to endure anything that comes your way. At this point, you become happy with who you have become and what you have created in your lifetime.

6. Find Absolute Certainty

It's perfectly okay to set goals beyond your present abilities or skills. What's important here is that you operate from a place of absolute belief and faith.

Frame your goals with absolute certainty—that no matter what, you'll find a way to make it happen. This is crucial for accomplishing your goals. Even if it seems impossible to you now, you know in your core that you can pull it off. When you have the fundamental belief, you will take back control of your life. So even though you may not be able to control the outside world or the challenges that come your way, you know that you'll persevere and overcome them.

So many people give up prematurely because they focus on the outcome and then stop and tell themselves "I don't know how to do that" or "I could never achieve that." Or they fail along the way and decide to quit because it seems easier than trying again. What if you didn't have to figure out how to get what you want, but rather believe that you will figure it out no matter what?

Achieving your goal is not only within the realm of possibilities, but it is an absolute certainty. Just imagine how that could change your life right now.

7. Deliberate Practice and Repetition

Repetition is the mother of skills. To master how to get what you want, you cannot set goals one time, never look at them again, and then expect long-term results. Your subconscious mind may know the general direction to move in, but the power comes from daily practice and constant review. People looking for a quick fix will never achieve mastery. Reaching your goals takes focus and deliberate practice. You must use your skills repeatedly to get what you want. In personal and professional settings, you must practice the skills of empathy and respect before you'll even be able to learn how to get people to do what you want.

If it's a new skill you want to acquire, you must practice and practice until you become comfortable in using it. If you're looking to achieve more in your business, then determine the core process you need to shift.

Mastering how to get what you want in life isn't easy. If it was, everyone would be joyful and fulfilled. Getting what you want takes time, commitment, and clarity of purpose. We are all capable of accomplishing the things we dream of; we simply must decide to go

Chapter Three : How to Fuel Success and Conquer Anything

after these goals with everything we have.

Are you ready to take control of your life and go after what it is you really want? Start today and set the future version of yourself up for success. Now that you have set your goals and you are ready to take control of your future, what you need to do next is to act.

Action Is the Key to Success

There is an enduring axiom of success that says, "The universe rewards action." Yet it is surprising how many people get bogged down in analyzing, planning, and organizing when what they really need to do is to act.

The question is: Will the powerful you turn on and start to act, or will you resist and wait just a little longer to get the joy, satisfaction, and fulfillment you deserve? Dreams and ambitions arise inside you as a signal, telling you that the powerful you should act right here, right now! The choice is always in front of you. Turn on the powerful you and move forward or give in to resistance and go nowhere. If you act, you can start to build momentum and roll your life in new directions towards something you want, such as to exercise regularly, to invest in stocks, or something that might make you feel happier about where your life is going.

It requires hard work and a commitment to succeed. You simply must develop a powerful mindset and push yourself to act, even when you don't like it. You must push yourself to do the things you don't want to do so you can become the person you were meant to be.

Always move from idea to execution as soon as possible. The longer your idea sits there, the less likely you'll act. Action unites body and mind. Every action starts with the inner mental impulse and finishes with a physical gesture that rubs you up against the fabric of the world. When you can act and see positive results, you feel powerful.

Don't try to find the right way to get started or you'll soon feel frustrated. Rather, push yourself to just start, without striving for perfection, and move forward and improve from there. You also should deal with all the uncertainty that surrounds your goal. You may have a hard time imagining exactly how you're going to achieve it. The world today is so complex and unforgiving. There is no instruction manual for life, and you probably don't have a network of knowledgeable and experienced people to help you break into something completely new. And it's true that the change you want to make is probably big, and the world doesn't let people cut to the front of the line with a smile. It takes real work to make things happen.

When you act, you trigger all kinds of things that will inevitably reward you with what you want. You begin to learn things from your experience that cannot be learned from listening to others or from reading books. You begin to get feedback about how to do things better, more effectively, and more quickly. Things that once seemed confusing become clear. Things that once appeared difficult become easier. You begin to attract others who will support and encourage you. All manner of good things begin to flow in your direction once you take action.

Move Like and with the Universe

The universe is alive with activity. There is movement all around. Nothing stands still, nothing stays the same, and everything is always in a constant state of change. If we want to work in accordance with the laws of the universe, we must move with the universe.

Nature seems to have a way to eliminate things that don't grow and don't move. Inaction and inactivity produce a vibe of decay, decomposition, and disease. Don't wait to make a move until you have mastered enough confidence. Paradoxically, life only becomes tiresome for those who avoid movement. An active mind and body remain invigorated. Act in life and life will act through you. Slow down life, and life will slow you down. Since the universe is full of activity, move, and

- Write that book

- Develop that app
- Act on that idea
- Start that business
- Implement that plan
- Use that gift
- Express that passion
- Fulfill that purpose
- Live that experience
- Magnify your life

Go Public with What You Want

You've now acted and are on your way to getting what you want to change your life. Now it's time to take your first step into the outside world and open your mouth and speak. The reason for going public is simple. Communicating is one of the most productive forms of action you can take. When you share your ideas, or ask someone for their help, you learn new ideas from others every time. And at the same time, you're advancing your own personal agenda and taking concrete steps towards your goals. Ask anyone who went through law school, and they will tell you that you can't really learn how to truly think on your feet without sparring with a partner. Preparedness and memorization count, but there's something else you learn when you rely on your verbal skills and perform a mock trial.

What is this something else? It's when we are forced to entertain an idea, and convey meaning in a persuasive manner, and juggle facts and rhetoric that our brains are challenged and we discover what we're capable of. It's a skill that must be acquired, and studies have shown that thinking on your feet lights up completely different parts of your brain. Speaking, defending, and explaining ideas offer a much tougher mental workout.

Simply put, talking about what you want will help you build the mental strength you need to get it. And just as important, by talking about your goals, you help make them real. When you sit around and think, "I should lose weight," you haven't really changed anything. But when you announce, "I'm going to lose weight," you enlist the outside world in holding you to your commitment.

There are three reasons why you cannot skip over this step.

- You can't get anything done in life without the help of other people.

- Other people accelerate your pace and broaden your ideas.

- Your relationship with other people is the most important aspect of your life.

You Need People to Get Stuff Done

Almost everything you do in life requires the help of others. To accomplish anything, you must ask for help. Asking is the world's most powerful and neglected secret to getting what you want. History is filled with examples of incredible riches and astounding benefits people have received simply by asking for them. Yet surprisingly, asking is still a challenge that holds most people back.

Ask repeatedly, because when you're asking others to participate in the fulfillment of your goals, some people are going to say no. They may have other priorities, commitments, or. The key is not to give up. Why? Because when you keep on asking—even the same person again and again you might get a yes. No wonder that the bestselling author Jack Canfield devoted an entire chapter on "Ask! Ask! Ask!" in his book *The Success Principles: How to Get from Where You Are to Where You Want to Be.*

Most people give up right when they're about to achieve success. They give up and quit at the last minute of the game, one foot from a winning touchdown. Persistence is probably the single most common quality of high achievers. They simply refuse to give up. The longer you hang in there, the greater the chance that something will happen in your favor. No matter how hard it seems, the longer you persist, the more likely your success.

B.C. Forbes, founder of *Forbes* magazine, was right when he said, "History has demonstrated that the most notable winners usually encountered heartbreaking obstacles before they triumphed. They won because they refused to become discouraged by their defeats."

Make a Positive Connection

The need to connect with other people is part of our genetic wiring. When you click with someone, you feel an instant rush. When you realize you have something in common, you start speaking faster and smiling without even realizing it. Even with a perfect stranger, if you smile enough and hold eye contact in a friendly way, you will feel a genuine bond with that person. I have experienced this many times with people who serve me coffee at a restaurant or people who share an elevator with me.

Scientists have discovered cells in your brain that are called *mirror neurons* that can copy the feelings, actions, and even sensations that another person feels. If someone else is smiling, you just can't help it, you must smile too.

You feel this urge to mimic in lots of ways. For example, you flinch when your friend cuts her hand slicing something. You can practically feel the knife scalping the tip of your own finger right off. That's your *mirror neurons* duplicating the sensations inside your own head. If you can't help but mirror the emotions, physical sensations, and actions of people around you, then you can use that to your advantage to help propel yourself forward and learn how to build an instant rapport with those people. This is part of why surrounding yourself with positive, motivated people is so important, because you'll be naturally inclined to mirror their emotions and behaviors.

Identify one person who has what you want or has done what you would like to try and reach out and ask that person for help. This person has tackled this mountain before you. He or she knows the terrain, the challenges, and the pitfalls. More importantly, he or she knows what *not* to do. This is the first shortcut to avoid losing time and money in trying to correct rookie mistakes. Your mentor also knows the short-cuts, the time-savers, the little tricks. You need a mentor.

Keep Up with Rapid Pace of Change

In today's world, a certain amount of improvement is necessary just to keep up with the rapid pace of change. New technologies are announced nearly every month! New techniques in industry are discovered even more often. And what we learn about ourselves and about the capacity for human thought continues almost unabated. Improving is therefore necessary to protect our achievements.

Whenever you set out to improve your skills, change your behavior, or better your family life or business, beginning in small, manageable steps gives you a greater chance of long-term success. Doing too much too fast not only overwhelms you, but it can also doom the effort to failure. When you start with small and achievable steps you can easily master, this reinforces your belief that you can easily improve.

To keep yourself focused on constant and never-ending improvement, ask yourself every day, "How can I improve today? What can I do better than before? Where can I learn a new skill or develop a new competency?" If you do, you will embark on a lifelong journey of improvement that will ensure your success.

If you make the commitment to learn something new every day, getting just a little bit better every day, then eventually, over time, you will reach your goals. Becoming a master takes time; you must practice, practice, and practice. You must hone your skills through constant use and refinement. It takes years to have the depth and breadth of experience that produces expertise, insight, and wisdom. Every book you read, every class you take, every experience you have is another building block in your occupation and your life.

Mastermind Your Way to Success

The concept of the "master mind alliance" was introduced by Napoleon Hill in his 1920s book, *The Law of Success*, and expanded upon in his 1930s book, *Think and Grow Rich*. While Napoleon Hill called it a "master mind alliance," it's been shortened and modernized to "mastermind group." Mastermind groups have been around since the beginning of time. Even Benjamin Franklin belonged to such a group, which he called the Junto. But it was Napoleon Hill who explained it clearly and encouraged people to gather in a structured, reputable environment for the success of all.

A mastermind group is like an objective board of directors, a success team, and a peer advisory group all rolled into one. Whether you find an existing mastermind group to join, or start a group of your own, you'll love what this group can help you accomplish.

The basic philosophy of a mastermind group is that more can be achieved in less time when people work together. A mastermind group is made up of people who come together on a regular basis to share ideas, thoughts, information, feedback, and resources. By getting the perspective, knowledge, experience, and resources of the others in the group, not only can you move beyond your own limited view of the world, but you can also advance your own goals and projects more quickly.

We all know that two heads are better than one, so imagine having a permanent group of five to six people who meet every week for the purpose of problem solving, brainstorming, networking, and motivating each other.

Mastermind groups also offer a combination of education, peer accountability, and support in a group setting to help build your business and sharpen your personal skills. The significance of a mastermind group is that it may include experts in systems used by millionaires. Every millionaire has systemized, streamlined, and organized the process of obtaining wealth. These mastermind group experts would bring in the most efficient form of information transfer that you'll learn and follow, whether you have chosen real estate, the stock market, or any other business.

Imagine what would happen when the combined force of mentors, teams, networks, or alternative energy and motor technologies experts seek solutions together? Miracles can happen in minutes.

Embrace Persistence

Once you embrace this principle of persistence, you will never fail. You'll add quality and riches to your life, eventually drawing you to the shores that your soul burns for. With this kind of rule, other people will view your efforts and accomplishments in amazement. This element will also produce a peace of mind that will never waver.

The challenges we face in life are exercises provided by nature. All development is the result of an effort, and this effort is what strengthens a person. Life favors those who can stick with things when the going gets tough, because it does get tough at times.

There has never been a successful or creative person who hasn't known failure, frustration, or tough times. Times when money was scarce or non-existent; times when he or she seemed out of touch with the rest of humanity; times when fresh ideas and inspiration didn't flow; and times when physical or emotional handicaps seemed insurmountable.

The hallmark of success is the ability to ride out these moments and still prevail. Frustration and disappointment, even sorrow, can lead to joy and prosperity. Often, those who overcome the fiercest difficulties are the men and women who ultimately achieve the greatest triumphs and inspire us the most.

Persistence is a characteristic of all men and women who have achieved greatness. It is not so much brilliance of intellect, talent, or resources as it is persistence of effort and constancy of purpose that draws greatness to the individual. Those who succeed in life are the men and women who keep the wheel turning, who do not believe themselves overly talented, but who realize that if they are ever to accomplish anything of value, they must do so with a determined and persistent effort.

When a persistent person undertakes anything, his battle is halfway over. Why? Because he or she will indeed accomplish all they are out to do. The persistent person never stops to consider the costs. Whether the major purpose leads them through mountains, over land, or across oceans, he or she must reach his or her goal dead or alive.

Greater than courage is persistence, the willingness to stand and keep trying. By determination, perseverance, and persistence, everyone should succeed in whatever they are doing. Once you get what you want in life, it's time for you to maximize your personal energy.

Maximize Your Personal Energy

Managing your personal energy is like managing the budget in a company. In business, every financial decision made in every department is connected. If the research and development group cuts spending today, eventually that decision will ripple through the organization and reduce profits in future years. Similarly, when you manage your personal energy, it is not enough to maximize it in the short run or in one defined area. Ideally, you want to manage your personal energy for the long-term and the big picture.

Maximizing your personal energy also means having something in your life that you are excited to wake up for. When your personal energy is right, the quality of your work is better, and you can complete it faster. That keeps your profession on track. And when all of that is working, and you feel relaxed and energetic and cheerful, your personal life is better too.

Matching Mental State to Productivity

One of the most important tricks for maximizing your productivity involves matching your mental state to the task. For example, when I first wake up, my brain is relaxed and creative. The act of writing is relatively easy because my brain is in exactly the right mode for that task. I know from experience that trying to be creative in the mid-afternoon is a waste of time. At 6:00 am, I'm a creator, and by 2:00 pm, I'm a copier.

Everyone is different, but you'll discover that most writers work either early in the morning or past midnight. That's when the creative juices flow more easily. When lunch time rolls around, I like to grab a quick snack and go exercise. At that time of the day, I have plenty of energy, so exercise seems like a good idea.

You might not think you're an early morning person. I didn't think I was either. But once you get used to it, you might never want to go back. You can accomplish more by the time other people wake up than most people accomplish all day. You're probably familiar with the term "body clock"—the mysterious guiding power responsible for making you sleepy at night and alert during the day in consistent twenty-four-hour cycles. You're probably also familiar with the fact that most of us don't abide by those clocks—we stay up late, drink coffee to stave off grogginess, and sleep in on the weekends. What you probably don't know, though, is that the key to unlocking your full potential is to get back in sync with your natural rhythm.

According to Michael Breus, the author of *The Power of When*, you shouldn't worry about *what* to do, or *how* to do it, but begin focusing on *when* to do it. You become more productive when your work is in sync with your natural rhythm.

Work Harder and Smarter

Everyone knows what working harder means, but what does working smarter mean? Often, working smarter means focusing on building

Chapter Three : How to Fuel Success and Conquer Anything

up a few of your strengths and doing away with a few weaknesses that really drag you down. An alternative approach is to find a team of people who substitute for the weaknesses that smart people have. Hard-working people don't build on their strengths.

When working on your goals, confidence, positive thinking, and hard work are all needed for achievement. Naturally, if you're taking on a larger endeavor, you'll need to put more effort and work into that too. It also pays to use your time wisely and more effectively to get things done quickly while reflecting on your achievements. What helped you achieve this goal in the first place? What method or approach did you take to make all of this happen for you?

Successful people in every field are often said to be "blessed with talent" or even lucky. But the truth is, many worked harder than the average person can imagine. From athletes like Michael Jordan to executives like Starbucks' CEO Howard Schultz, these people are known for waking up early and working towards a goal while other people are still in bed.

Michael Jordan had prodigious physical gifts. But as his long-time coach Phil Jackson writes, it was hard work that made him a legend. When Jordan first entered the league, his jump shot wasn't good enough. He spent his off-season taking hundreds of jumpers a day until it was perfect.

Since returning to turn around the company, Schultz gets into the office by six in the morning and stays until seven in the evening. Anyone can do it. Let these people be an inspiration. During the 1980s and 1990s, I worked like Michael Jordan and Howard Schultz and surprised the management and the board of directors of the Panafric Hotel in Kenya's capital, Nairobi. When I joined the hotel as a sales representative, the room occupancy was at 35 percent of its capacity. Six months later, the occupancy had increased from 35 to 65 percent. It was at this time the managing director nicknamed me the Miracle Man, thanks to my qualifications in sales, marketing, and public relations, combined with hard and smart work.

The time came when we didn't have any rooms available because the hotel was full almost all the time. At this time, I was promoted to the managerial position of a sales executive with the powers and privileges to use my signature as a form of currency while promoting the hotel.

Sitting Position

Your brain takes some of its cues from what your body is doing. My experience is that when I sit in a position I associate with relaxation, such as slumping on the couch, my brain will start the lazy relaxation subroutine. But if I sit with good posture, both feet on the floor, my body signals to my brain that it's time to concentrate on work.

Consistency might be more important than the specific position you choose. If you train yourself to concentrate when you're sitting on the couch with your laptop, that might become a good place for you to work. Just don't make the mistake of using the same sitting position for work that you use for relaxation. If the couch is where you choose to nap or watch television, it will probably be a poor place for doing serious work.

Tidiness

Tidiness, in my personal experience, has an impact on your energy. Every second I look at a messy room and think about fixing it is a distraction from my more important thoughts.

I realize that clutter and messiness don't affect everyone the same way. Some people need to have things just right, and others don't seem to mind living in chaos. My experience is that after straightening up my office and working through piles of miscellaneous tasks, I feel more clearheaded and energetic. I don't assume my experience is universal, but the cause and effect in my case is so strong that I do recommend you experiment with it. All you need to do is pay attention to how you feel after you have tidied up your workplace compared with how you felt when it was a mess.

Cleaning and organizing your space is boring work, and you might never see it as a priority. One trick I've learned is that I automatically generate enthusiasm about tidying up if I know someone is stopping by. That's why it's a good idea to invite people over on a regular basis. It will inspire you to keep your place straightened up, and that might in turn cause your mind to have a bit more energy.

Don't Fear, Ask

One of the biggest obstacles to success, and a real energy killer, is the fear that you don't know how to do the stuff that your project requires. For example, you might have a terrific idea for a small business, but you don't know how to register a name, how to do your accounting, how to build a website, how to outsource work in a foreign country, and so on.

When you don't know anything about a particular topic, it's easy to assume it would be too hard to learn it quickly. Don't be afraid to ask. When you start asking questions, you often discover that there's a simple solution, a website that handles it, or a professional who takes care of it for a reasonable fee. Keep in mind that every time you wonder how to do something, a few hundred million people have probably wondered the same thing. And that usually means the information has already been packaged and simplified, and in some cases sold. But it's often free for the asking.

I'm a big fan of flash research, the type you do in less than a minute using Google. You might think a topic is too complicated to master, but you might learn otherwise in less than a minute if you bother to check. I'm routinely surprised that someone else had the same question and left a simple breadcrumb trail for me to follow.

I can't think of a single instance in which I was stopped because I couldn't find the information I needed. I think most entrepreneurs would tell you the same thing. And more to the point of this chapter, when you know how to do something you feel more energized to take it on.

Prioritize

You need to get your priorities right so the things you love can thrive. The biggest priority is you. If you severely harm or damage your health or situation, you won't be able to focus on any of your other priorities. So, taking care of your own health is priority number one. Your second is your lifelong learning, while your third biggest priority is economics. That includes your job, your profession, your investments, and even your house. You might wince at the fact that I put economics ahead of my family, my friends, and the rest of the world, but there's a good reason. If you don't get your personal financial engine working right, you place a burden on everyone from your family to the country. Your fourth and final priority is your community, your country, and the world, in that order.

The Joy of Living

Once you achieve what you want in life, you've reached the climax and the finish line of your effort. You must also learn for your own benefit, and for those who love and depend on you, how to deal with success once you have achieved it. And this is usually a more difficult challenge than any you have faced while you were struggling to reach the pinnacle.

Clearly money is a great thing, but it's not everything. Money can buy temporary happiness, but not everlasting life. Even family, health, friends, and spiritual values are more important because they constitute true wealth. Money is an energy tool. Money can build or destroy. In his popular book, *The Art of Living*, Norman Vincent Peale urges us to slow down and take the time to live, because success without the joy of living is a game for fools.

When Mrs. Ramsay MacDonald, wife of a former British prime minister, was dying, she called her husband to her bedside for a last word. "Keep romance in the lives of our children," she admonished him.

Chapter Three : How to Fuel Success and Conquer Anything

It was an impressive parting message, which, as we reflect upon it, is deep wisdom. This mother knew, as all who meditate seriously upon life must know, that the passing years make a terrific assault upon the zest of man's spirit, and unless he exercises care, will steal from him the romance of life. Napoleon Bonaparte said, "Men grow old quickly on the battlefield," and they do in life also, unless they are vigilant.

Popular essayist Charles Lamb once said, "Our spirits grow gray before our hairs." One starts out in youth with anticipation, excitedly looks towards the approaching years with the spirit of an adventurer, but before he has traveled far, life starts blowing its cold winds upon him. He tries his wings, but they fail him. This is one of the saddest things that can happen to anyone, to lose the thrill and zest of living. The romance of life is so priceless a possession that it is a supreme tragedy to lose it. Though one may acquire much in wealth, fame, or honor, the real joy of life doesn't lie there, but rather, in keeping the romance of living going. Nothing gives such complete and profound happiness as the perpetually fresh wonder and mystery of life.

What frightens me is that men and women are content with what is not life at all. We pass hastily through life restless, hurried, anxious, and call it living. Deep in our hearts, however, we know that real life is better than that; it is a great and wonderful experience which is to be fervently desired.

We have been made to believe that to live rich, we must be rich. But you know what? It's simply not true. Life doesn't start when you've got a lot of money in the bank. The truth is that your life is on the right track because it has already started, and to live rich is to know what makes you happy when you're at home, with friends and family, and finally, in your relationships.

Peace of mind is one of the best things that you should enjoy in your life. Napoleon Hill tells us a fascinating story of his visit with John D. Rockefeller Sr., the oil magnate and the world's richest person at that time. During their meeting, Rockefeller asked the young reporter if he would like to change places with him. Without hesitation Hill politely told him that he would not, that he valued his health and freedom—

neither of which Rockefeller, for his opulence, had or enjoyed.

Today, this hectic, hurrying age of ours has left the average man and woman bewildered and out of breath. It has made us think that the greatest virtue is to keep up with the ticking clocks. We seem to have the idea that everyone must be constantly doing something. People all over the world, including you and me, need to reduce life's tempo or else we'll allow this hurly-burly digital age to rob us of life's deepest meaning and happiness.

Let us take time to live and enjoy life because we are not machines.

A Word of Wisdom

Living and enjoying the success of the day while thinking about the future is an art to be learned. There is no room for complacency. There is always the next level to aspire to or the assurance of the success you've achieved through improvement, personal growth, and development. It's easy to become complacent after reaching a level of accomplishment. Success is not a one-time event. It's something to be worked for in an ongoing capacity. Always reflect on where you've come from. What are the things that worked for you? Why did they work? You need to answer these questions to ensure your unshakable success in the future.

CHAPTER FOUR

Money Mastery

Since time immemorial, nothing man has ever invented has received so much attention, is so widely sought and has generated so much controversy as our paper and coin money. It is both used and worshipped. Some say that it liberates people, others say that it enslaves them.

The desire for material gain is fundamental in human nature. Men and women have been concerned about prosperity and wealth since the first coin was fashioned in Asia Minor around 750 BC. Many human beings have said that money is like good health and most of them are concerned if they don't have it. True happiness consists not in the possession of things, but in the privilege of self-expression using material things. You must have money to enjoy freedom of body and mind.

It's Your Right to Have Money

Money is a great motivator. Increasing your net worth, accumulating wealth to help others, and earning money for the advantages it can offer you and your family are worthwhile objectives. The availability of money frees your mind to concentrate on achieving your goals. If you know that your expenses are covered and you are relieved of the worry that comes with paying your debts, you can devote all your time and energy to achieving your objectives.

There's also a peace of mind that comes with financial security that allows you to set your own agenda for your life. You no longer have to haggle over unexpected expenses that could throw your business or family budget into a tailspin. A healthy cash reserve is the best protection against financial ruin.

Wealth is neither physical nor limited. Wealth takes on contrasting forms—vision, discipline, work, faith, initiative, resilience, desire, ideas, and thought—all unlimited and infinite. Wealth's most salient characteristic is that it's available to all and is primarily *metaphysical—not physical*. Consequently, the creation of wealth lies within you, the individual. If you skipped reading my life story after arriving in Canada, go back and learn how I made money in stocks when I was about to turn sixty-five.

Understanding the Rules of Money

Most people do not have a proper understanding of the rules of money, even though they are playing money's game by having an income and expenses. But like other games, you need to understand the rules if you want to win. If you want to properly handle and use money, you must learn basic money management skills.

In chapter five, you will learn all about lifelong learning for people who are no longer raising a family, as well as how to learn the right knowledge or become tech savvy. So, if you want to master money management, there is no age limit.

Another thing to understand about money is budgeting. Unless you set a budget and follow it religiously, you will not achieve your goals. It's easy to skip this step, but remember, you need money to make money. Budgeting means allocating your money into specific pools for recurring basic expenses, discretionary spending, and future savings and investments.

Money Grows When We Spend Less Than We Earn

Those who really desire to attain independence have only to set their minds upon it and adopt the proper means, as they do about any other objective, and the thing is easily done. But however, making money is not as hard as keeping it.

Many people understand simple economics, and they know economy is wealth. They know they can't have their cake and eat it also. If you agree that keeping money is more difficult than spending it, please follow this advice: Wear the old clothes a little longer if necessary; dispense with the new pair of gloves; mend the old dress; live on plainer food, if need be, so that under any circumstances, unless some unforeseen accident occurs, there will be a margin in favor of income. A penny here and a dollar there, invested at interest, goes on accumulating, and in this way the desired result is attained.

It requires some personal discipline to always be conscious of your spending. When you get used to this positive habit, you'll find there is more satisfaction in rational saving than in irrational spending. If you find that you have no surplus at the end of the year, and yet have good income, you should buy a small notebook and write down every item of expenditure daily or weekly in two columns, one headed "necessities," and the other headed "luxurious. When this is done, you'll find that the latter column will be double, treble, and frequently ten times greater than the former.

Dr. Benjamin Franklin said, "It's the eyes of others and not our own eyes which ruin us. If all the world were blind except myself, I would not care for fine clothes or furniture." Ladies and gentlemen, you need not go to the trouble of pretending. Don't try to look smart like your neighbor or spend as much as she or he spends because you are not as rich as he or she is.

If you continue to pretend and waste your time and spend your money foolishly to keep up appearances and impress people, you will be deceiving nobody but yourself.

Some older adults accustomed to gratifying every whim and caprice will find it hard, at first, to cut down their various unnecessary expenses, and will feel it's a great self-denial to live in a house smaller than they have been accustomed to, with less expensive furniture, less company, less costly clothing, fewer parties, theatre-goings, pleasure excursions, cigar-smoking, liquor-drinking, flying first class, and other extravagances. But, after all, if they try depositing a small sum of money, at interest or judiciously invest in land, they'll be surprised at the pleasure to be derived from constantly adding to their little "pile," as well as from other economic habits such as saving and vulgarity.

Some families expend thousands and thousands of dollars per annum, and would scarcely know how to live on less, while others secure more solid enjoyment frequently on a small part of their income. Many people, as they begin to prosper, immediately expand their ideas, and commence expending for luxuries, until in a short time their expenses swallow up their income, and they become ruined in their ridiculous attempts to keep up appearances and be recognized.

Money is in some respects like fire—it's a very excellent servant but a terrible master. When you have it mastering you, when interest is consistently piling up against you, it will keep you down in the worst kind of slavery. But if you let money work for you, then you will have the most devoted servant in the world. There is nothing animate that will work so faithfully as money when invested at interest, well secured. It works day and night, and in wet or dry weather.

Today the amount of consumer debt amassed by an average household in some countries is staggering. Add to that consumer debt a mortgage payment, car payment, not to mention daily groceries and other necessities purchased on credit cards. They commit what little money is left over each month to pay off past purchases rather than to investing for their future lifestyle.

Smart people, on the other hand, have mastered the spending game. They live below their means. They pay less for what they need. And they figure out how to accomplish what they want to do while spending as little as possible. Spending too much can wreak havoc with your financial goals. It keeps you in debt, prevents you from saving as much as you can, and turns your focus to consumption, rather than to wealth creation and accumulation.

Stay Active, Make Money, and Strive in Old Age

Believe it or not, plenty of jobs for older people are available. And yes, you can work after retirement—for all kinds of good reasons. For example, maybe you want to earn extra money, help others, meet new people, or explore something profitable you've always dreamed about but never had the chance to try before. Or maybe you've heard that, as you grow older, having a job can provide a surprising number of benefits for your physical and mental health.

Retirement used to mean the end of your working life, but having a job during one's senior years is now becoming increasingly common.

It's not surprising that employers now actively look forward to hiring seniors. More and more of them are starting to recognize that experienced and mature workers often have strengths that some younger workers lack. Out of all age groups, workers over the age of sixty-five demonstrate the highest levels of positive engagement on the job.

Are you a writer and subject matter expert? If you are, another way to share your knowledge is by writing about it. In this age of information, many people are looking for authoritative content online or in print. So, if you're an expert on a particular subject, get your name out there! Begin by starting a blog, publishing articles on platforms such as LinkedIn, or approaching publications related to your area of expertise.

If you've been a teacher, why not teach others about your field?

Community colleges and community centers often hire temporary instructors to teach classes for professional development or general interest. So, check out your local college, community center, or seniors' center to see what's already being offered and inquire about the possibility of creating new classes based on your area of expertise. Keep in mind that you don't have to be an academic scholar or professor. Your knowledge and experience could be enough to qualify you to teach self-enrichment classes in a college's continuing education department.

Aside perhaps from some extremely physically demanding occupations, almost any job that can be done by a younger person can be done by someone older depending on the individual. In other words, the best jobs for older workers vary according to each person's goals, capabilities, and health.

The following jobs are arranged by what may be driving you to seek employment:

- You want to stay involved in a prior career field.
- You want to get out and about in your community.
- You want social contact.
- You want to help people.
- You want to make money and receive good benefits.
- You want to work at a job that isn't physically challenging.
- You want to stay active because you're in good shape.
- You want to get a job related to a favorite hobby.
- You want to be a consultant.

Customer Representative. Do you enjoy talking on the phone? Why not help people by answering questions and solving problems? You need patience and good communication skills for this job. Basic computer knowledge is also required but working-at-home jobs are also available.

Tour Guide. Are you good with history and geography? This job will give you an opportunity to share your love of local attractions and inspire others with your knowledge. Depending on the venue, you could meet people from around the world. Public speaking skills and a good memory are essential.

Retail Salesperson. This is one of the most popular jobs for seniors. And it's easy to see why. Retail positions often have flexible schedules, opportunities for friendly contact with customers, and you could work at a store that aligns with your personal interests. A bookstore would be a good place for you if you like to read, a clothing store if you follow fashion, or a sporting goods store if you're athletically inclined.

Administrative Assistant. Your role would be to help businesses and organizations run smoothly by answering phones, booking appointments, responding to customers' questions, and doing other administrative tasks. This work is often done sitting down. However, you need vision for most positions.

Virtual Assistant. These workers do tasks like those of administrative assistants, but they typically work remotely. So, this is a great option for seniors who are looking for jobs at home as the work can be done anywhere with a good Internet connection.

Tax Preparer. Are you good at doing your own taxes? Why not make some money by preparing tax returns for other people? You don't have to be a certified accountant, but you do need to obtain a Preparer Identification Number from the IRS or the CRA if you're an American or Canadian, respectively. For other countries, you can find out what is needed to become a tax preparer.

Pay for Every Purchase with Cash

One way to save is to start paying with cash for everything. Cash is more immediate. It makes you think about what you're buying, and you'll probably find yourself spending less than you would if you used credit cards. Every potential purchase will be more carefully considered as "necessary," incidentals will become less necessary, and large purchases will probably be put off, forcing you to think about how you can make do without them.

Eliminate Unnecessary Daily Expenses

It's never too late. Starting today, consider adding up the cost of all the unnecessary things you've been spending money on and compare that amount to what you could be spending that money on—either depositing it in your mutual fund, enjoying rich and rewarding life experiences, or paying for things that are much more critical to your happiness. Wouldn't a vacation, a personal development opportunity, or a health club membership make life more enjoyable and inspire you to achieve financial growth?

David Bach, bestselling author of *Start Late, Finish Rich*, calls this prudent strategy the "Latte Factor"—the idea that if you eliminate small but unnecessary daily expenses, such as that $4 cup of morning coffee from the gourmet coffee shop or hitting the mall for retail therapy you could redirect the savings into investments that would help achieve your financial goals. While these expenses might seem small, it always surprises people how quickly they add up to substantial savings.

Avoid Being in Debt

Another way to increase wealth is to avoid being in debt by adopting a less consumerist lifestyle. Credit card, mortgage, and auto payments are staggering for many people. If you are one of those whose savings and financial security are shaky, take steps now to start living a debt free life. Here are some ways to do so:

1. Prioritize Your Spending

Any time you want to buy something, ask yourself if the item you have in mind is essential or unnecessary. Essential things are those which you can't survive without, such as food, water, shelter, sleep, safety needs, health, or love. You can't survive without all these things. If you're an asthmatic patient, then an inhaler is a must buy. If you are diabetic, you're obliged to spend money on special foods that don't increase the glucose in your body.

For non-essential things, you can still find ways to spend less on them. Fly economy, instead of first class, don't buy an expensive sofa set to impress your visitors, or spend a lot of dollars on your birthday party.

2. Gradually Increase Your Debt Payments

As soon you pay off a smaller debt, simply take the monthly payment you were making on that debt and use it to increase your payment on your next debt. Here's an example. If by paying $400 a month on your credit card you reduce your balance to zero, take that same $400 next month and add it to the amount you would normally pay on your car loan. This is likely to save you thousands of dollars in interest by paying off your car loan early, plus it keeps you from expanding your lifestyle by that $400.

3. Settle Your Smallest Debts First

When you settle your smallest debt, you achieve a major success breakthrough—even if it doesn't seem that way. When one goal is accomplished, you experience a huge boost in your self-esteem. It also makes you more motivated to settle another debt, if any.

Live Beneath Your Means

Living beneath your means involves waiting until you have the money before you buy something. This gives you the benefit of avoiding borrowing and paying interest charges. It also gives you a waiting period during which you may well discover that you don't want those intended things after all. The prudent side of living beneath your means is that you'll use and enjoy what you have and harvest a full measure of fulfillment from it, whether it is your old house, your steamboat, or your old suit. It also means that you can cope with the economic bad times when they come—which they will.

Take Care of What You Have

Our bodies are the most common and important thing that we all want to last as long as possible. Paying attention to proven preventive practices will save you lots of money. Taking care of your blood circulation, for instance, can save thousands on blood pressure medication. And eating healthy may save you thousands in expensive procedures—not to mention it may save your life.

Extend this principle to all of what you own. Replace your computer's old hard drive, repair your worn shoes, mend your torn clothes, and renovate your small old house. Regular oil changes are known to extend the life of your car and dusting your refrigerator coils conserves energy and could save your appliance.

Many of us have lived with excess for so long that it no longer occurs to us to maintain what we have. But more costs money and may not be available in the long run. We need to rewrite our brain to think *repair rather than replace*.

Wear Out Everything You Own

If it weren't for the fashion industry, we could all enjoy the same basic wardrobe for many years. Are you upgrading or duplicating last year's phone, furniture, kitchenware, and linens, or are you truly using them up? Think how much money you would save if you simply decided to extend the use of things over 25 percent longer. If you usually buy new bedding every three years, try replacing them every four years. If you trade in your car every four years, try to extend that to five. If you buy a new coat every other winter, see whether every third winter would do just as well. And when you are about to buy something, ask yourself, "Do I already have one of these that is in perfectly usable condition?"

Before trashing something, ask yourself whether there might be another way to use part or all of it. Old and worn-out clothing become cleaning rags. Old magazines become art materials. The web is full of creative do-it-yourself hacks that can help you reuse everyday items.

If your car is taking you for a ride, costing more money in repairs or more hours in tinkering than it is giving you in service, buy a new one. If your knees are suffering from running shoes that have lost their bounce, it would be cheaper to buy a new pair than to have knee surgery.

Consider What You Need Before Buying

Forethought in purchasing can bring significant savings. With enough lead time you will likely find items you need at a cheaper price. Keep a list of things you expect you'll be needing soon. Get to know the brands, features, and typical price ranges for those items. Use the tools from your favorite deals' sites, online retailers, or classified advertising sites like Craigslist, Kijiji.ca, or eBay to receive notifications when the item you need becomes available or changes price. Being ready to pounce on a deal will ensure you get the item at the sale price, since many of the best deals are gone in days, hours, or even minutes. Watch seasonal bargains around major holidays, especially at stores that still advertise in local newspapers.

By anticipating that you'll run out of milk this week, or noticing that the expiry date of your bread is approaching, you can purchase them during your supermarket shopping instead of running out to the expensive corner store to pick up these items. This can result in significant savings over the long term.

Research Your Purchases

Take notice of reviews, comments, and ratings from trusted sites and online marketplaces when you are doing your research. You should decide what features are most important to you. Don't buy the cheapest item available. Durability might be critical for something you plan to use daily for fifteen years. The smart way of saving money is to spend less on each item you buy, but it's equally true that spending $50 on something that lasts seven years instead of buying a $20 one that will need to be replaced in four years will save you $30.

You can also evaluate quality by developing a sharp eye and carefully examining what you are buying. Are the seams in a piece of clothing ample? Are the edges finished? Is the fabric durable? Are the screws holding the appliance together sturdy enough for the job? Is this material strong enough? Is this table nailed and properly screwed? You will become an expert materialist—knowing materials so well that you can read the probable longevity of an item the way a forester can read the age and history of a fallen tree.

Comparison-Shopping and Bargaining

Another smart way to spend less is to buy used. After all, most of us live in used houses. Since a vehicle loses 20 percent of its purchase price once it leaves the car showroom, if you buy a car that is a few months old, you can save thousands of dollars. Like cars, furniture loses its value quickly, so buying a mint-condition sofa, or a used dining set on Craigslist, will certainly save you good money.

Thrift stores have been fashionable emporiums for a long time. Clothing, kitchenware, furniture—all can be found in thrift stores, and you may be surprised at the quality you can find in many of them. If you just can't bring yourself to shop at thrift stores, consider *consignment stores*. The prices are higher, but the quality is often higher as well.

Meet Your Needs with Substitutes

There are hundreds if not thousands of ways to meet your needs. Economics would have you believe that more, better, or the other stuff can satisfy almost any need and is just a click of a button away. Don't make the mistake that frugal pleasures are less enjoyable because they are less costly. What do you usually do to feel good when you are down? Maybe you enjoy listening to music, watching a movie, getting a massage, or retail therapy? Maybe you need a change of scenery? You are going to choose what strategies work best for you.

Remember, substitution is a frugality strategy. It isn't about lowering your traditional standard or downgrading pleasure. It's about ensuring that I get precisely what I'm seeking for less, or nothing at all. I'm not limiting myself; I'm letting go of rigid standards. Substitution isn't deprivation; it's about getting creative and smarter with your money.

Spending Money Wisely

Spending money wisely basically means getting the most for your money in line with what matters to you. In turn, this puts you on the path to achieving your financial goals. An essential part of personal finance is knowing how to spend your money and avoiding financial traps that won't let you out of that rut.

Having a budget is also a key to wise spending. Making a budget is the most important thing you can do to manage your money, but many people are reluctant to take this beneficial action because they associate budgeting with restrictions, and a lot of hassle and headaches. Or you may feel like you do not make enough money to warrant a budget. However, budgeting is essential because it can help you save, eliminate overspending, and enable you to make the most of every dollar.

Budgeting stops overspending. Spending money without thinking carefully about where it's all going can easily lead you to overspend every month. When you use budgeting in your personal life or business, it puts you in control. It allows you to prioritize your spending, track how you are doing, and realize when you need to make changes. A budget puts a solid plan into place that is easy to follow and gives you the chance to plan and prepare for the future.

One method financial experts recommend using when trying to reach a financial goal is the "50/30/20 budgeting rule." Through this strategy, you allocate your budget according to three categories: needs, wants, and savings. This way, you will be setting aside money each month for your goals.

Budgeting is not about limiting the fun in our lives; it's about opening up opportunities to have more fun and worry less about our financial safety. By categorizing your budget, you will be able to see where everything is going and have fewer reasons to be anxious about future expenses.

You can simplify the budgeting process by using percentages of your income for set expenses, spending money, and savings. Then you simply track the money as you utilize it. The first few months of budgeting are a bit more difficult as you work to find the amounts that are appropriate for your situation. If you have a friend or partner who is interested in getting a handle on their finances, consider making a budget together. This way, you can hold each other accountable, making the process easier and more fun.

Now that we have a clear idea of how budgeting translates into wise spending, let us learn how investing your money is a great and wise way to spend your cash.

Invest a Portion of Your Money Every Month

Spending your money wisely entails not only eliminating unnecessary expenses but also putting the money you saved into activities that can help you achieve your financial objectives. Another great way to spend your money wisely is to invest it. Like self-improvement, money you spend on investments is more so an investment in your future as opposed to an expense. If you don't have much money to invest every month, that's completely okay, but everyone can afford to invest a little, even if you are living paycheck to paycheck. Thanks to compounding interest, you'd be very surprised at how much a little bit of money can accumulate into a big range of investments over the course of a few years.

Not only is investing your money a wise move financially, but you'll probably be happier too knowing that your financial future is looking bright.

Bad Spending Habits to Avoid

Here are bad spending habits you must avoid at all costs:

1. Eating Out Frequently

Do you find yourself buying lunch and ordering in more than a couple of times a week? Well, let's say the cost of lunch is $10 a day. Multiply that by five days a week for one year and we are talking $2,400 in takeout!

How to spend that money wisely? Cut back on buying lunch by a third or by half and put the money you don't spend towards savings or paying off debt. You'll be surprised how much you save when you cut back. Plus, you can free up extra money for your grocery budget and buy some of the nice foods you've always wanted to try out. Combine that with meal planning and not only will you save a ton of money, but you'll also be aware of the nutrition of everything you are eating because you picked out the ingredients and cooked it yourself.

2. Buying Coffee Every Single Day

Are you one of those people who needs that morning coffee fix? Do you find yourself stopping at Tim Hortons or Starbucks too many times a week? Or even multiple times a day? Well, depending on where you buy your coffee, you can very well be spending an average of $4 a day for a single cup. Over one year that's $1,460!

How to spend that money wisely? Consider investing in your own fancy at-home coffeemaker. It might seem a big investment, as good ones can range anywhere from $100 to $400, but if you are a big coffee drinker, you'll be saving a lot of money by making your own coffee at home. And over time, your homemade coffee will come out to pennies compared to an average of $4 a day.

3. Paying ATM Fees

Have you ever withdrawn from an out of network ATM and thought to yourself, "It's a $3 fee, it's not that much"? Well, if you do this once a week or four to five times a month at an average of $3 per out of network withdrawal, then we're talking $180 in ATM fees a year.

Wouldn't you rather put that money to better use? It could go towards your savings, a vacation, your emergency fund, or be used to treat yourself to something nice.

How to spend that money wisely? Open a checking account with a bank that has no ATM transaction fees regardless of what ATM you use, or one that reimburses out-of-network ATM fees. You can also make sure to pull out enough cash from your in-network ATM based on how much you think you'll be spending each week, and you can determine that by creating a budget.

4. Paying Late Fees

While this is not a spending habit, it can be indirectly related to not having enough money to pay bills on time, which is related to your spending. If you've ever paid a late fee, you know it sucks to have to pay extra. Late fees are usually excessively high and, if unexpected, can cause other issues like bank fees due to insufficient funds.

In many instances, late fees average around $25, and if you are paying a late fee even just once a month multiplied by twelve months is a whopping $300! Yuck!

How to spend that money wisely? Set reminders on your calendars for your bills and their due dates. This will help you to be aware of all your upcoming bills and expenses. You can also call up your service providers or creditors and ask them to move your due dates to be closer to the dates when you get paid; that way you can plan to pay your bills right away.

5. Buying Things You Don't Use

If you were to check in your closet right now, how many clothes do you have with the tags still attached or that you planned to wear but you never got around to or perhaps wore just one time? It's common for people to spend a lot of money on clothes, shoes, and accessories just to show off.

Good Spending Habits to Embrace

The following are easy and frugal habits that will have a positive impact on your finances:

1. Sell What You Don't Use

Before your next shopping trip, take some time to clean out your closet to get rid of what you don't wear or don't need. Consider selling these items to make extra money, and then donate or give away the rest.

2. Buy Things You Know You Will Use

Next, make a list of all the gaps in your closet. Basically, the things you need but don't have and the things you wear often but have gotten worn out or too old and use that list as a guideline the next time you go shopping so you are buying things you know you will use.

3. Include Shopping in Your Budget

Finally, build your shopping into your budget and create a collection of clothes that you would normally need to wear. Yes, it's okay to shop and buy nice things, but you want to make sure you can afford what you're buying and that it's not at the expense of your financial goals or obligations.

4. Travel During the Off Season

Whether you're going to Rome, Tokyo, or New Delhi, each vacation has a different peak travel time. So, do your research and figure out when the off season starts in your vacation spot. You may not come back with plenty of photos, but you'll save hundreds of dollars on airfare and accommodation.

5. Go Meatless

The price of meat is generally high in most countries. So, try to incorporate more meatless meals into your diet. You don't have to become a full-time vegetarian but consider making meat more of a side dish than an entrée. There are lots of tasty meatless meals you can enjoy at a fraction of what the meat version would cost. Search Google, Pinterest, or Allrecipes.com for endless ideas.

6. Focus on Things You Value

Money management is all about learning from your mistakes and using them as opportunities to reorganize your finances. Your money should be used for four things: savings, investing, enjoyment, and giving. These are four practical areas to spend your money that will lead to building not only wealth, but an emergency fund for those unexpected life events.

Giving to others is also a key to building wealth and experiencing enjoyment from doing so. These are some tips for spending money in a practical and meaningful way.

7. Don't Buy Liabilities

Consider the long-term advantages and disadvantages of the purchases you're making. Many transactions are impulsive decisions to buy something you don't need, or simply need to intimidate someone you don't like. So, while this is fine when purchasing a chocolate bar at the supermarket, it becomes a bit of a challenge when you're out shopping for cars and trying to impress your neighbors. Consider how anything will benefit you in the future before you buy it. How long do you think it will last? Is it going to put you in unnecessary debt or is the benefit you'll get out of it over the course of its life worth the price?

8. Learn to Value Savings Over Products

Some people are born with the ability to make and save money while others regard money as something that must be spent as soon as it is in their possession, and anything else is a waste of time. If you fall into the second category, you should strive to adopt a mindset that prioritizes savings over purchases. In the end, money invested and saved will almost always improve your life more than money spent on things that you won't be interested in in the future.

You need to start thinking about what you can do with the money you're saving, or you'll never save anything. And it's at this point that knowing how to spend your money wisely becomes important, because it leads to an increase in your income.

9. It's Better to Pay for the Quality

Many people buy things that are cheap but poor in quality. We usually don't feel the impact of cheap things right away, but if we need to replace them after six months or a year, we might be paying more than what we would have paid if we were buying quality things. That's why I do my research before I go shopping, ensuring the product I'm buying has good reviews.

With that said, this doesn't apply to everything. For example, buying an expensive vehicle won't save you money in the long run. But buying high-quality, durable clothes that will last you for several years, now that's money well-spent.

10. Add Value to Your Home

Another practical and beneficial way to spend money wisely is to add value to your home through repairs and renovations. Whether repairing a leak or installing a new wardrobe, upgrading your home in subtle ways will allow you to spend your money prudently and have a higher value and better-looking home.

11. Creating a Roadblock Against Spending

So how do you create a roadblock?

- Leave your wallet at home when you're just going for a walk near the local shopping center, where you may be tempted to buy something on impulse.
- Empty your wallet and pay yourself first by depositing that little money into your retirement and savings accounts, so you remain without money readily available.
- When you want to buy something, ask yourself if you can afford it, or if it is necessary. Consider why you really wanted the thing in the first place and how it fits with your goals.

12. Learn from Warren Buffett, the Wisest Money-Spender Billionaire

You might want to live like a billionaire—but only if that billionaire is Warren Buffett. This investor, known as the Oracle of Omaha, is the CEO of Berkshire Hathaway. But there is more to this American business magnate than just his job.

Despite his roughly $116.7 billion net worth as of 2022, and being the fifth wealthiest man in the world according to *Forbes*, Buffet enjoys a life of simple taste, frugal living, and generous philanthropy. Have a look at how exemplary he is.

- **Warren Buffett's house is the same one he bought in 1958.** Billionaires live in mansions, right? Not Buffett. He lives in the same residence in Omaha, Nebraska, he bought in 1958 for $31,500, the equivalent of roughly $285,000 in 2020. Buffett has no intention of putting his home up for sale. "I wouldn't trade it for anything," he told CNBC earlier in 2021. In today's money, Buffett would have paid about $43 per square foot for the 6,570 square foot home. But in 2021, the home was worth about $161 per square foot, according to the home's current value listed by the tax assessor's office in Douglas County, Nebraska.

If you want to live like Buffett, consider buying a smaller home than you can afford. Instead of paying pricey mortgage payments, you will be able to put more of your money towards savings, retirement, or vacations.

- **Buffett starts the day with a cheap breakfast.** You might assume billionaires have their brunch at the most extravagant restaurants, or they employ a personal chef who can whip up whatever they want whenever they want it, right? Wrong. Adopting Buffett's lifestyle doesn't include paying high prices for daily gourmet French toast prepared in the comfort of your own home. When it comes to food, the billionaire investor has been known to save money by taking the fast-food route.

- **Buffett buys reduced-price cars.** Although some CEOs drive around in million-dollar cars, you'll likely find Buffett driving something much more modest. In a BBC documentary, his daughter, Suzie Buffett, said he bought cars that he could get at reduced prices like those that had been damaged by hail. The cars were fixed and didn't look hail-damaged and became a regular part of Buffett's lifestyle. "You must understand, he keeps cars until I tell him. This is getting embarrassing—it's time for a new car," his daughter said in the documentary.

  Remember this next time you're in the market for a car. As I mentioned earlier, cars tend to depreciate quickly, so it is better for your finances if you try to keep your well-working car for as long as possible—or at least opt to buy a used car instead of new.

- **Buffett enjoys affordable hobbies.** Committing to live like Warren Buffett doesn't mean all work and no play. After all, billionaires have hobbies. But compared to other famous CEOs, investors, and entrepreneurs, Buffett's hobbies are much more affordable. For example, he enjoys playing bridge. "If I play bridge and a naked woman walks by, I don't even see her," laughed Buffett during a CBS News-*Sunday Morning* interview. Yep, Buffett is a self-proclaimed addict, playing the game about eight hours a week, according to a 2017 *Washington Post* interview.

When Buffett is not busy being a business mogul, you might find him strumming his ukulele and singing as well. He has played for investors and charity events. A video of him playing the instrument with Bill Gates even went viral after it was posted on Gates's blog in 2016.

- **Buffett treats his friends well, but not extravagantly.** What do you give to a friend who is also a billionaire? Buffett's long-standing friendship with Gates is legendary. In honor of Buffett's ninetieth birthday, the Microsoft magnate explained on his blog what's kept their friendship strong over the years: "Of all the things I've learned from Warren, the most important might be what friendship is all about," Gates wrote. "A person that I admire as well as like—that's the perfect description of how I feel about Warren. Happy birthday, my friend." In his 2016 blog post, Gates gave examples of how Buffett is a kind and thoughtful friend, such as driving personally to the airport to pick up Gates whenever he's in Buffett's hometown, calling frequently, and sending news clippings by mail that he thinks Gates and his wife will enjoy.

- **Buffett used a Nokia flip phone long after smartphones existed.** Buffett likely won't be spending big money on the newest iPhone, even though he's now using one. The billionaire revealed in a February 2020 CNBC *Squawk Box* interview that he has been given several iPhones, including

Chapter Four : Money Mastery

by Tim Cook, and was using the iPhone 11 at the time. If you insist on buying the latest iPhone to hit the market, look for other ways to save on your phone expenses, such as using a non-contract phone plan or buying a family plan to share data.

- **Buffett doesn't splurge on designer suits.** Buffett shuns high-end designer suits. Instead, he exclusively wears suits created by a Chinese entrepreneur named Madame Li Guilian, whom he met in 2007. "They fit perfectly," he said of the suits in a 2017 CNBC interview. "We get compliments on them. It has been a long time since I got compliments on how I look, but when I'm wearing Madame Li Guilian's suits, I get compliments all the time."

    The takeaway: You should opt for quality goods that will last you a long time, rather than buying something just because it has a brand name attached to it.

- **Buffett clips coupons.** Buffett proves that even billionaires still appreciate an opportunity to save money. In Bill and Melinda Gates's 2017 annual letter, Bill recalled a trip he took with the investor, during which Buffett paid for their fast-food lunch using coupons. He even provided photographic proof. "Remember the laugh we had when we traveled together to Hong Kong and decided to get lunch at McDonald's? You offered to pay, dug into your pocket, and pulled out coupons!" Bill wrote. "It reminded us how much you value a good deal."

    The takeaway: Save on your next purchase—even if it's something as inexpensive as a McDonald's meal, by using coupons, which you can easily find online.

- **Buffett has worked in the same office for more than fifty years.** Buffett has remained in the same office building since he joined Berkshire Hathaway in the 1960s. "It's a different sort of place," Buffett said of the company's Omaha headquarters in the 2017 HBO documentary *Becoming Warren Buffett*. "We have twenty-five people in the office, and if you go back, it's the same twenty. The exact same ones. We don't have a public relations department. We don't have a general counsel. We just don't go for anything that people do just as a matter of form."

The takeaway: Even if you're not a business owner, you can still benefit from Buffett's way of thinking. It boils down to the old saying: "If it isn't broken, don't fix it."

- **Buffett thinks outside the box to save money.** In Roger Lowenstein's biography of the businessman, *Buffett: The Making of an American Capitalist*, the author says that after Buffett's first child was born, he converted a dresser drawer into a space for the baby to sleep instead of spending money on a bassinet. When it came to the second child, he borrowed a crib rather than bought one.

    Perhaps making your baby sleep in a drawer seems a little extreme, but it's just an example of thinking outside the box. Use the resources that are already available to you to prevent unnecessary spending.

- **Buffett values relationships over material things.** Buffett explained his choice to live frugally during a Q&A session he conducted with a group of business school students. "You can't buy health and you can't buy love," said Buffett, according to the *Underground Value* blog. "I'm a member of every golf club that I want to be a member of [...]. I would rather play golf here with people I like than at the fanciest golf courses in the world. I'm not interested in cars, and my goal is not to make people envious," he told *People* magazine in 2017.

    Suzie Buffett said of her father: "It's true that he does not care about having a bunch of money. Instead, he emphasizes family. I don't think people realize he's got a bunch of great-grandchildren, and he could tell you everything about what they're all doing. He knows every one of those kids, and he knows about their lives."

You Better Be Selfish

To save for success, you'll find yourself continually trying to balance your own needs with the needs of others. You'll always wonder if you're being too selfish or not selfish enough. My experience has taught me that there are three kinds of people in the world.

- Selfish
- Stupid
- Burden on others

Your best option is to be selfish, because being stupid or a burden on society won't help anyone. Society hopes you'll handle your selfishness with some grace and compassion. If you do selfishness right, you'll automatically become a net benefit to society. Successful people generally don't burden the world. Most successful people give more than they personally consume, in the form of taxes, charity work, job creation, and so on.

Successful people don't cause worry and stress for those who care for them. As a successful person, you can be a role model for the right kind of selfishness.

Spend Your Money for Maximum Happiness

To spend your money as wisely as possible, try to maximize your happiness with every dollar you spend. What I mean is that you should try to avoid spending money on things that don't add much to your life. For example, if you love to travel more than anything else, then spend your money on vacations.

So be proactive and spend your hard-earned money in a way that makes you happy. No one is here to tell you what makes you happy, all I'm saying is don't feel bad about spending money (even overspending) on things that add true value to your life.

Our culture of consumption expands exponentially, and our lives increasingly revolve around money—earning it and saving it. What most experts can agree on is that there are ways to spend our money that are more likely to elicit joy. So next time a commercial has you itching to pull out your wallet, hit pause and consider where to invest your cash. You can spend it on saving time by hiring people to do your most dreaded tasks, from scrubbing toilets to cleaning gutters. This way money can transform the way we spend our time, freeing us to pursue our passions.

Yet wealthy individuals do not spend every day in happier ways; thus, they fail to use their money to free themselves. Research suggests that people who think of their time as a limited resource are more likely to derive joy from life's simple pleasures, like eating sweets or talking to a friend.

If you can afford to hire someone to clean your house, do it. Buying time is a great investment because it allows us to pursue things that we find meaningful and enjoyable. A universally hated activity is commuting. People regard it as a stressful waste of time. But it allows you to enjoy nature and improve your fitness while walking to and from bus stops and workplaces.

Even spending time on simple, low-cost pleasures, like drinking cold beer with friends, can produce small, frequent boosts in mood and facilitate social connections. Even investing in a fancy bottle of wine during a Zoom happy hour, or in outdoor recreation, is money well spent.

Another way of maximizing your happiness is to contribute to the well-being of others. This is because we are rational beings through and through. By making a positive difference in someone's life we derive a sense of pride and satisfaction. We help and get recognized for it. This is a good investment.

Chapter Four : Money Mastery

Good Financial Management for Every Older Adult

It's important to remember that sustaining healthy finances as a senior often requires taking some special factors into consideration. For example, your goals for the immediate and more distant future are probably very different from what they were a few decades ago. You may also have close relatives who want to help you, who need financial assistance of their own, or who may inherit your assets. Plus, you can't ignore your health care needs, or the fact that protecting your money becomes increasingly important as you age.

Be realistic. And be specific. Remember to consider fun things like your hobbies, leisure activities, and potential travel.

You should also keep in mind that, as you age, you may need elderly care or assistance with certain aspects of everyday living. Do your goals reflect that possibility and consider how you'd like to be cared for if you experience health challenges? Map out a vision of what you want for the rest of your life. Doing so can help you avoid some of the pitfalls that other seniors experience. By re-establishing your goals and reviewing them on a frequent basis, you'll create a more solid foundation from which to build greater financial security and life satisfaction.

Identify every source of incoming money that you can reliably count on. Are you receiving social security? Do you have income from a pension? What about income from investments such as certificates of deposit, stocks, bonds, or mutual funds? Is it possible that you'll outlive your money? Many people underestimate how long they'll live. As a result, they withdraw their savings too quickly and end up with unexpected changes to their lifestyles. You might live longer than you think. Are you prepared for that? Did you save every penny for a rainy day and housing in old age? If you did, congratulations!

The Financial Situations of Older Adults

Since housing is typically the single largest item in a household budget, housing affordability has important repercussions for overall well-being. For homeowners, housing can also be an important source of wealth, one that can be tapped to pay for home modifications needed to age in place. And when a household reaches the stage where they need additional services to continue to live independently, their ability to pay for such services will depend significantly on their housing situations and costs. Not surprisingly, older adults' financial resources vary widely.

While many older adults are secure, able to cover the costs of housing, other necessities, and long-term care if needed, significant numbers of low, moderate-income households live in unaffordable housing and lack the assets to cover the costs of home modifications or in-home support. Going forward, if current income and wealth distributions hold, population and household growth among older ages will mean millions more older owners and renters in precarious financial situations.

Housing Cost Burdens

In 2014, 78 percent of households headed by a person aged sixty-five and older owned their homes, while the remaining 22 percent were renters. Monthly housing costs vary widely by tenure and mortgage status: in 2014, the median monthly costs for homes owned outright by a person aged sixty-five and older were $450; for renters, $770; and for owners with a mortgage, $1,262, largely reflecting these significant differences in costs, the shares of older households that are housing cost burdened, paying more than 30 percent of gross income towards housing costs, are closely linked to tenure type and presence of a mortgage. Owners aged sixty-five and over who own their homes outright are least likely to be housing cost burdened (17 percent), while more than half (55 percent) of renters of the same age bear housing cost burdens.

Income and Wealth in Combination

Given the differences in wealth described above, large disparities exist between the total financial reserves of owners and renters. Even excluding owners' home equity, the typical older renter household has substantially lower income and wealth than the typical older owner. Sixty-seven percent of renters aged sixty-five and older bring in less than $30,000 per year and hold under $50,000 in net wealth, compared with 23 percent of owners of the same age. The number of renters with very low financial reserves is more than double the number with middle-to-high financial reserves: one-quarter (24 percent) of all renters aged sixty-five and older hold less than $5,000 in non-housing net wealth, and have an annual income under $15,000 per year, while just 11 percent of older renters bring in at least $30,000 in income and hold at least $150,000 in non-housing net wealth. Older owners, on the other hand, are far less likely to be at risk of financial security in later life, even without cashing in the valuable safety net of home equity.

Several trends may reshape the financial realities faced by older households in coming decades. These include an increase in prevalence and median amount of housing debt carried by older households, and a rising median income and labor force. If the current cost burden rates by age and tenure hold constant, by 2035, the number of older adult households alone will probably double.

I truly hope that if you are between fifty-five and sixty-four, the above information is a wake-up call for you. You still have plenty of time to invest, using the services of financial planners and financial advisors. For those who are sixty-five and above and have some financial reserves, financial experts can advise you how to invest in non-risky portfolios. Talk to Professor Google to learn where these financial experts operate from.

CHAPTER FIVE

Global and Personal Lifelong Learning

Global lifelong learning is an international movement whose aims are the education and stimulation of the many retired members of the community—those in their third age of life. Its original conception, which began in France as an extramural university activity, later spread to other European countries, the United States, Australia, Asia, and Canada.

The "third age" is defined as a time in your life (not necessarily chronological) where you can undertake learning for its own sake. There is no minimum age, but a focus on people who are no longer in full-time employment or raising a family.

Universities of the third age do not issue diplomas, but rather certificates, and teach in many fields according to the interests of the older students (usually over fifty-five). Some of the subjects taught are computer skills, languages, entrepreneurship, hereditary law, religion, and politics.

The Third Age Network (TAN) is very active in Canada, however, currently only within the province of Ontario, with their head office at the G. Raymond Chang School of Continuing Education at Toronto Metropolitan University. The network started in 2007 and has grown to twenty-one groups in 2018.

The Third Age Network's mission is "To foster Third Age Learning and share issues and solutions to common organizational challenges. We do this by promoting the establishment of organizations that provide opportunities for older adults to learn in a friendly, social setting and by supporting adult learning organizations in this process by sharing strategies and techniques to accomplish this goal."

Why did I choose this topic for this entire chapter? Because I am a student of lifelong learning. Since my young age I read every single day. I lived in Kenya in my early thirties and began investing in government bonds in my forties, thanks to reading about the success of Warren Buffett, the greatest investor of all time. If I didn't read every day, I wouldn't have managed to write this book comprising different topics, but with one common theme—success.

What Is Lifelong Learning?

Lifelong learning is automatic, which means we see things, we observe them, and then learn something new through our experiences. So, it's a continuous process and a lifelong one. Lifelong learning can be intentional, conscious, or unconscious, for better or for worse.

Lifelong learning is all learning activity undertaken throughout life, with the aim of improving knowledge, skills, and competences with a personal, social, and occupational perspective. It's learning that occurs after the formal education years of childhood, where learning is instructor driven or pedagogical, and into adulthood, where learning is individually driven and andragogical. It is sought out naturally through life experiences as the learner seeks to gain knowledge for professional or personal reasons. These natural experiences can come about on purpose or throughout life's unpredictable course.

Chapter Five : Global and Personal Lifelong Learning

It's through lifelong learning that Warren Buffett, Bill Gates, Barack Obama, and Benjamin Franklin developed their intelligence, and got to where they are today.

Key Differences Between Lifelong Learning and Education

Lifelong learning is a process that results in relatively long-lasting changes in the individual's behavior by way of training and experience. On the other hand, education is a systematic process of imparting or gaining knowledge, developing the basic skills of reasoning and judgement, and preparing an individual to live a matured and mannered life.

Lifelong learning is a natural or coincidental process where a person learns many things daily, which is not purposeful. In contrast, education is deliberate in the sense that one has a clear idea of the fact that they are being educated by enrolling in a course or attending an institution.

A lifelong learning process means that there is no age barrier to learn something; even at the age of ninety one can learn how to cook, how to sing, or how to play a game. But in the case of education, people of different age groups can enroll themselves at an institution to receive an education.

How to Adopt Lifelong Learning?

1. Recognize your own personal interests and goals because lifelong learning is about you, not other people and what they want. Reflect on what you're passionate about and what you envision for your own future. If progressing your profession is your personal interest, then there are ways to participate in self-directed learning to accomplish this goal. If learning history is your passion, there are likewise ways to explore this interest further.

2. Make a list of what you would like to do or be able to do. Once you've identified what motivates you, explore what it is about that particular interest that you want to learn.

3. Identify how you would like to get involved and what resources are available. Achieving our personal goals begins with figuring out how to get started. Researching the interest and goal will help to formulate how to go about learning it.

4. Structure the lifelong learning goal into your life. Fitting a new learning goal into your busy life takes consideration and effort. If you don't make time and space for it, it won't happen. It can easily lead to discouragement or quitting the learning initiative altogether. Plan out how the requirements of this initiative can fit into your life or what you need to do to make it fit. For example, if learning a new language is the goal, can you make time for one hour a day? Or does fifteen minutes a day sound more realistic? Understanding the time and space you can devote to the goal can help you to stick with the goal in the long run.

5. Make a commitment. Committing to your decision to engage in a new lifelong learning initiative is the final and most important step. If you've set realistic expectations and have the self-motivation to see it through, commit to it and avoid making excuses.

How to Learn the Right Knowledge?

So how do we learn the right knowledge and have it pay off for us? You can follow the following steps:

1. Identify Valuable Knowledge at the Right Time

The value of knowledge isn't static. It changes depending on how valuable other people consider it and how rare it is. As new technologies mature and reshape industries, there is often a deficit of people with the needed skills, which creates the potential for high compensation.

Because of this high compensation, some people are quickly trained, and the average compensation decreases.

2. Learn and Master That Knowledge Quickly

Opportunity windows are temporary in nature. Individuals must take advantage of them when they see them. This means being able to learn new skills quickly. After reading thousands of books, articles, and magazines about this topic, I've found that understanding and using mental models is one of the most universal skills that everyone should learn. It provides a strong foundation of knowledge that applies across several fields, so when you jump into a new field, you have pre-existing knowledge you can use to learn faster. I recommend reading *Mental Models: How to Improve Your Life, Make Better Decisions and Avoid Cognitive Biases with Strategic Thinking and Mental Models* written by Dave Thorniley.

3. Communicate the Value of Your Skills to Others

People with the same skills can command widely different salaries and fees based on how well they're able to communicate with others. This ability adds value in different ways to existing skills you already have. Many people spend years mastering an underlying technical skill and virtually no time mastering this multiplier skill.

4. Convert Knowledge into Money and Results

There are many ways to transform knowledge into value in your life. A few examples include building a successful business, selling your knowledge as a consultant, and building a reputation by becoming a thought leader.

5. Learn How to Financially Invest in Learning to Get the Highest Return

Each of us needs to find the right "portfolio" of books, online courses, and certificate or degree programs to help us achieve our goals within our budget. There is little to no difference between investing in knowledge or finance, because we expect a return on investment in both choices.

6. Master the Skills of Learning How to Learn

Mastering the skills of learning how to learn increases the value of every hour we devote to learning—or learning rate—which determines how quickly our knowledge compounds over time.

We must shift our focus to a more savvy and realistic quest for knowledge. Just as we have minimum recommended dosages of vitamins, steps per day, and minutes of aerobic exercise for maintaining physical health, we need to be rigorous about the minimum dose of deliberate lifelong learning that will maintain our economic health. The long-term effects of intellectual complacency are just as insidious as the long- term effects of not exercising, eating well, or sleeping enough.

As I've just said above, we must shift our focus to a more savvy and realistic quest for right knowledge, and you should start by becoming tech savvy if you truly want to make your life richer.

Becoming Tech Savvy Is All You Need

Seniors in a digital world can be easily overwhelmed by new technology. We are surrounded by smartphones, social media, tablets, banking machines, or laptops. There is no avoiding it, so we should learn how to use all these technological advances to make our lives easier. It's easy to become a tech-savvy senior when you begin to learn more about the technology around you.

You live in a time unlike any other. Your parents and ancestors did not have the tools that you have at your disposal. If they wanted to change their lives, it took a lot of money, a new degree, and very probably a move across the country. In practice, most of them didn't have a chance in hell of changing anything. They were stuck in the same job, the same circle of friends, and the same town for most of their adult lives.

Chapter Five : Global and Personal Lifelong Learning

But the world has changed enormously since then. Unlike your parents, you have exactly what you need to get what you desire. Because of technology, the proliferation of information on the Web, hyperconnectivity, and oversharing through social media, you have access to everything you need. There's a way to get whatever you want without requiring money, a degree, or a cross-country move. And no matter how crazy, far-fetched, or scary your desire feels, there is someone on the planet who has done it and has probably published about it, been featured in some magazine, or joined an online group to help them get it done. There is a living, breathing example of the life you imagine out there right now, and you are going to use that person and all the tools at your disposal to help yourself get that life.

What is so exciting, but also daunting, is that while anyone connected to the Internet has access to more information than ever before in history, this kind of access has also created a problem. There is so much information to choose from. Because of this overwhelming quantity of resources, succeeding in the digital age requires a more diligent approach to time management, information management, and life management. If you are not careful, you can end up lost in irrelevant information. Information is useful, but it is the information you act on that makes a difference to your success.

One of the truly life-changing aspects of the digital age is that the Internet gives talented people the ability to work from anywhere if they have a computer and an Internet connection. Not only has this created a massive shift in how, when, and where people work, it has given rise to an entire workforce of remote workers, flex-time workers, outsource vendors, and virtual assistants.

In addition to bringing us knowledge and connections, the digital age has endowed us with a vast army of technological devices and self-improvement tools that help make us smarter, help us to never miss an appointment, let us research and work with coaches, find mentors and partners, and learn new skills. There are over a million apps for your smartphones that teach us about anything you want to learn. And there are dozens of apps that help you develop a success mindset. It's an amazing time to be alive and the perfect time to thrive. Imagine how blessed we are! Most devices are designed to do multiple things. Look at what smartphones help us to do today. We can also attend classes, make videos, watch TV, and read e-books on our tablets. Our laptops and desktop computers can do even more.

Today, technology is used in every facet of life because it provides the speed, connectivity, and efficiency to make tasks easier. We all want things to be easier, and as an older adult, it's important not to underestimate how technology can help you in your golden years. This is the information age where questions can be answered in an instant, and when we take advantage of being informed and connected, then we can gain the knowledge and know-how necessary to help ourselves and improve our lives. With digital literacy training, older adults can gain the skills and confidence to access information and services online.

Indeed, getting some simple training in using computers, tablets, and smartphones can help seniors to stay connected with their families, friends, and communities. This is especially important for seniors who wish to live independently and age at home.

Here are examples of useful things you can do with a computer:

- Browse the Internet
- Use email
- Manage your finances
- Play games
- Download and watch movies
- Listen to music
- Stay in touch with friends and family via social media sites such as Facebook or communication software like Skype.
- Share photo albums!
- Edit your own videos and photos

Whether you want to learn how to use email, browse the Internet, have video calls with your grandkids, purchase gifts or other items online, or share and view photos with friends and family, it's easier than you think.

If you have a family member (grandkids are naturals!) or a friend to show you some basics, that's great. If not, then there are several choices out there. Where do you start? Good news! There are lots of resources for seniors who want to know their way around computers and be able to improve their ability to survive in the digital age.

How-To Books for Seniors

Visit your local library or bookstore. There you'll be sure to find a variety of books to help you learn how to use different types of technologies. Some are quite simple to follow and written specifically for seniors, such as Visual Steps and the *For Dummies* series. You can also order these books online at sites like Amazon.com, Barnes & Noble, Better World Books, and many more.

Online Instruction

If you already have access to a computer and can use the Internet, then there are several online services that offer technology lessons and instructional videos while allowing you to go at your own pace.

The first resource is GCFLearnFree.org, which is free of charge and supported by the Goodwill Community Foundation. Another free website that teaches seniors basic computer skills is TechBoomers.com.

The Connecticut Distance Learning Consortium's "Basic Online Skills" tutorial is a short, simple introduction to basic computing in about an hour, new computer users can learn how to use a mouse, save files, access a CD-ROM, open and close software files, and copy and paste files or text. If you don't mind doing a bit of browsing, there are also many YouTube video instructors who can offer quick overviews on general computer know-how and specifics such as setting up a Facebook account or doing Skype calls.

Take a Local Class or Workshop

You will probably be able to find a local workshop or class for seniors right in your own community. Indeed, there is a great demand for such types of courses. Whether it's a beginner's class for computer basics or a specific series on how to become proficient using certain software or applications, it's a great way to get out and learn with peers.

Other Important Things You Can Do Because of Lifelong Learning

If you are searching for your next job or volunteer opportunity, **Idealist.org** can help you get comfortable using online search tools and filters. Since 1995, Idealist.org has been connecting people and organizations to help build a better world. Currently over 1.5 million individuals have created accounts, and hundreds of thousands opt to receive free email alerts when new listings are posted that match their areas of interests and geographical location. All these services are also available in Spanish and Portuguese.

Virtual volunteering offers opportunities to support causes you're passionate about and gain computer experience at the same time. Virtual volunteering is done online, via computers, tablets, or smartphones, usually off-site from the non-profit organization being supported. More and more organizations are engaging people who want to continue their skills and volunteer their time via the Internet. Virtual volunteering is flexible, often allowing the volunteer to complete a task or project on their own schedule. It is also not limited by geography, physical ability, or work arrangement. You can choose to volunteer for an organization in your local community, across the country, or across the globe, all without needing to leave your home.

LinkedIn is the world's largest professional network on the Internet. You can use LinkedIn to find the right job or internship, connect and strengthen professional relationships, and learn the skills you need to succeed in your occupation. You can access LinkedIn from a desktop or your phone via a browser or app.

A complete LinkedIn profile can help you connect with opportunities by showcasing your unique professional story through your experience, skills, and education. You can also use LinkedIn to organize offline events, join groups, write articles, post photos and videos, and more.

Who should be joining LinkedIn? LinkedIn is a platform for anyone who is looking to advance their profession. This can include people from various professional backgrounds, such as small business owners, students, and job seekers. LinkedIn members can tap into a network of professionals, companies, and groups within and beyond their industries.

The **AARP Now App** delivers senior-specific news, shares local events, and lets you know of any discounts you may qualify for within an AARP membership. Also check out AARP Back to Work 50+. If you live in Canada, CARP, formerly the Canadian Association for Retired Persons, is Canada's largest advocacy association for Canadians as we age. CARP's mission is to advocate for better healthcare, financial security, and freedom from ageism (age discrimination). If you live outside the United States and Canada, you can find an equivalent association in your own country.

Evernote is a free app for your smartphone and computer that stores everything you could possibly imagine losing track of, like a boarding pass, receipt, article you want to read, to-do list, or even a simple typed note. This app works brilliantly, keeping everything in sync between your computer, smartphone, or tablet.

Senior Net is a 501(c) (3) non-profit organization specializing in computer and Internet education for adults fifty-five and over and those in need. In addition to providing education to older adults, Senior Net furnishes computer skills and education to veterans, the underserved, disabled, and those with impairments.

Silver Surf is a free app for iPhone and iPad that features large navigation buttons and allows users to zoom in on text and set higher contrast to make viewing easier. It is intended for individuals over the age of fifty who utilize the Internet on a consistent basis.

Technology for Seniors Made Easy is a Facebook group offering tips and information for working and managing life online.

Trello is an online project management app that lets you set deadlines, assign tasks, and have conversations with colleagues. It gives you a simple way to see a project through to completion.

Benefits of Lifelong Learning

Whether pursuing personal interests and passions or chasing professional ambitions, lifelong learning can help us to achieve personal fulfillment and satisfaction. It recognizes that humans have a natural drive to explore, learn, and grow, and encourages us to improve our quality of life and sense of self-worth by paying attention to the ideas and goals that inspire us.

But what does personal fulfillment mean? Personal fulfillment and development refer to the natural interests, curiosities, and motivations that push us to learn new things. We learn for ourselves, not for someone else. The reality is that most of us have goals or interests outside of our formal schooling and jobs. That is part of what it means to be human; we have a natural curiosity, and we are natural learners. We develop and grow, thanks to our ability to learn.

Lifelong learning recognizes that not all our learning comes from classrooms. For example, in childhood, we learn to talk or to ride a bike. As adults, we learn how to use a smartphone or how to cook a new dish. These are examples of everyday lifelong learning we engage in daily, either through socialization, trial and error, or self-initiated study.

The benefits of lifelong learning go beyond professional advancement. It can help you understand how the world works. It can help you realize your passions and boost your creativity. The world of work is rapidly changing, and people need lifelong learning to advance their skills and stay relevant.

In his book *Learn or Die*, Edward Hess cites today's increasing globalization and rapidly evolving technologies as reasons that individuals and organizations must maximize their ability to learn, since learning is the foundation of continuous improvement, operational excellence, and innovation.

Lifelong learning increases the abilities of seniors who have always wanted to run a business to do so in retirement. It can be an opportunity to develop entrepreneurial skills. In fact, starting a business is a popular way for retirees to make some money while enjoying the benefits of being their own boss. People in the fifty-five to sixty-four age group start new companies at a high rate in many countries.

Even though we might think of start-ups as the domain of younger people, many older adults are also well-suited for entrepreneurship. Your ambitions for this stage of life may go beyond simply having enough money to meet your basic needs. Whether you want to travel the world or do something else that matters to you, with the right business, you can fund those goals.

Being an entrepreneur adds more money to your lifelong earnings, which raises the amount of social security you're eligible for. And if you're making enough money, you can probably delay applying for Social Security. Your benefits will increase for every year you work past retirement age, until you turn to a certain age in your own country. Again, if you managed your savings wisely, a few more years of growth could add up to a substantial amount.

CHAPTER SIX

Embrace Humor for Happiness and Success

The use of little Humor can help us become happier, healthier, and make our lives richer. Humor is an essential and learnable skill that everyone needs to build a great life that all of us deserve.

Humor is shown to be fundamental to our success as a species. The financial benefits of a good sense of humor are so profound that colleges such as Stanford University are offering business courses on humor in the workplace. The big goal is to teach students how to achieve business objectives, build more effective and innovative organizations, cultivate stronger bonds, and capture more lasting memories. It doesn't stop there, though. Stanford Graduate School of Business professors believe humor has the power to make and scale positive change in the world.

All of us, therefore, embrace humor to infuse or inspire the kind of humanity, humility, and intellectual perspective that only humor can bring. If you make humor one of your frontline passions, you will be amazed by how it will enrich your life. Haven't we all been influenced by someone's passion? Imagine what can happen when a strong sense of purpose is fueled with passion? There is no doubt that a healthy sense of humor can help you achieve greater results at an individual, team, and organizational level.

Humor has the power to transform experiences, ideas, and people. "Humor is not only a connector, and a builder, but also a catalyst. It has the potential to make our lives richer," says Michael Kerr, author of *The Humor Advantage*. All this is possible if you use humor effectively. Make sure the humor you use laughs with the people, not at people. Use humor to tear down walls of indifference and build social and economic bridges.

Always remember that being humorous is about being more human, having a bigger heart and demonstrating greater humility. During uncertain times, what people need most is a good laugh. Imagine what would happen if all of us understood there is an untapped force contained within us that has the positive power to totally change our lives. And what if we discovered all we had to do to unlock this secret weapon was simply to start using it?

Mark Twain was right when he said, "*Humor is the great thing, the saving thing after all. The minute it crops up, all our hardnesses yield, all our irritations, and resentments flit away, and a sunny spirit takes their place.*" Humor may very well be the great thing. It touches upon nearly every facet of life. Studies and surveys report that men and women find a sense of humor is the most important quality in a partner. So, don't hesitate to embrace it.

There are three main theories of humor from which you can choose to use one or two. **Relief theory** argues that laughter and humor are ways of blowing off psychological steam, a way to release psych energy. That's why jokes told at funerals are often met not with the silence that a somber occasion like that would merit, but with uproarious laughter instead.

Superiority theory was originally formulated by Plato and Aristotle to explain a specific kind of humor: why we laugh at others' misfortunes. In this theory, humor is a means of declaring one's

Chapter Six : Embrace Humor for Happiness and Success

superiority over others. If you are looking to cultivate a sense of humor to improve your leadership and likeability skills, this is not the kind you want to acquire.

Incongruity theory argues that humor arises when two contrasting, distinct ideas are mingled. Humor often subverts expectations, and punchlines are often the results of an unexpected reversal. Consider Oscar Wilde's "Work is the curse of the drinking classes"—it's funny because it both reverses a common phrase and because it subverts a more conventional way of looking at the world.

Humor Is a Learnable Skill

Comedians need both talent and training to succeed. But too many people are under the impression that humor is an innate ability, not a skill you can learn. In other words, we tend to believe we're either funny or we're not. Researcher and psychologist Carol Dweck says that domains once thought to be wired into our genetic coding, like intelligence and creativity, are not fixed. We can change them by adopting what she calls a *growth mindset*. Humor is not some binary feature of our genetic code, but rather a skill we can strengthen through training and use, much as we would strengthen our leg muscles by working out at the gym, climbing stairs, and walking around neighborhoods.

There are courses in humor techniques at The Second City—the World's Premiere School of Comedy. That's where comedy experts Anne Libera and Kelly Leonard trained talents like Stephen Colbert, Steve Carell, and even some talents like Tina Fey, Chris Redd, and Julia Louis-Dreyfus. You, too, can develop a sense of humor.

Why Humor Is a Key to Success

"If we couldn't laugh, we would all go insane."—Robert Frost

Whenever tough times sweep in, humor follows behind. This is true during the Coronavirus pandemic.

After closing from visitors, the prestigious British Royal Academy of Arts issued a "ham drawing contest" that resulted in a bizarre display of ham drawing prowess across the country (a ham hunched over a desk working, a set of Dali hams resembling the famous melting clocks painting, and even a tattoo of a ham on one man's thumb). In true comedic form, comedians Sam Morrill and Taylor Tomlinson moved in together and began producing an entire comedy show called "New Couple Gets Quarantined." There is also a *New York Times* therapist who shared in her article that more and more of her patients take virtual therapy calls seated on the toilet to ensure privacy. One, she said, even had a breakthrough when they accidentally bumped the flusher mid-conversation and laughed for the first time in a month. The list of strange, funny, and complex responses to social distancing could honestly be a book in and of itself.

To state the obvious, jokes like these happen during difficult times, because they make us feel good. They pull us away from negative thinking and into a more positive space. In the workplace especially, humor and a lighter environment benefit people and companies far beyond the moment of laughter.

Humor builds teams. When the British Royal Academy surprised everyone with the ham challenge purely for the sake of fun, people responded with surprisingly creative takes. The same thing happens on the team level at organizations. Research shows that teams that joke and approach work in a playful manner build solidarity, trust, and a safe atmosphere where people feel they can be creative and genuine. The result is that each team member feels empowered, less tied down to a strict hierarchy.

Humor has been researched as the source for positive results within a productive and successful workplace. Decrease of absenteeism and employee turnover, increased productivity and levels of innovation and creativity are some of the outcomes when humor is intertwined within a workplace culture.

Chapter Six : Embrace Humor for Happiness and Success

Research conducted by Harvard Business Review noted a positive correlation between senior executives practicing humor in the workplace and their bonus levels. Other researchers suggest that most effective and highest rated leaders also have a positive sense of humor.

Humor strengthen bonds between people, create rapport with customers, get and hold attention, strengthen memory of the points you want to be remembered, persuade others to see (and perhaps adopt) your point of view, make awkward communications less difficult, deflect criticism, reduce tension, frustration and anger, manage conflicts, reduce burnout, remove intimidating barriers between management and non-management employees, bolster eroding trust, boost morale and motivate employees, build resilience, stimulate problem solving, sustain a positive attitude on the job, and keep everyday hassle and problems in perspective.

People who use humor tend to be more approachable. The more approachable you are, especially as a leader, the honest and open people tend to be, the more successful and innovative teams tend to be. Humor can help companies and to stand out and go beyond with their customer service, garnering them a huge loyal following.

Many companies have experienced tremendous results by effectively putting humor to work. If you are in business, don't get sucked into thinking that humor can't work for you. The truth is that "More Humor = More Money" is at an individual, team, and organizational level.

A good number of surveys suggest that humor can be at least one of the keys to success. A Robert Half International survey, for instance, found that 91 percent of executives believe a sense of humor is important for career advancement; while 84 percent feel that people with a good sense of humor do a better job. Another study by Bell Leadership Institute found that the two most desirable traits in leaders were a strong work ethic and a good sense of humor.

Companies such as Zappos and Southwest Airlines have used humor and a positive fun culture to help brand their business. You don't have to be a stand-up comedian, but well-placed humor that is clever and apropos to business situations always enhances an employee's advancement. While you are still working or not, humor is likely to help you in whatever you're engaged in life.

Here are 8 additional reasons why humor is a key to success at work:

1. **People will enjoy working with you.** People want to work with people they like. Why wouldn't you? You spend huge chunks of your working hours at work, so you don't want it to be a death march. Humor deftly employed is a great way to win friends and influence people. You need to be funny, but not snarky (that is not good for team building) and you can't offend anyone.

2. **Humor is a potent stress buster.** In fact, it's a triple whammy. Humor offers a cognitive shift in how you view your stressors; an emotional response; and a physical response that relaxes you when you laugh.

3. **Humor is humanizing.** Humor doesn't build hierarchal walls, but bridges that allow all people to come together, realizing that we all seek common ground.

4. **It puts others at ease.** Humor is a way to break through the tension barrier. Research shows that humor is a fabulous tension breaker in the workplace. People who laugh in response to a conflict tend to shift from convergent thinking where they can see only solutions, to divergent thinking where multiple plays with ideas are considered.

5. **Ha + ha = Haha!** Humor is a key ingredient in creative thinking. It helps people play with ideas, lower their internal critic, and see things in new ways. Humor and creativity are both about looking at your challenges in novel ways and about making new connections you've never thought about before.

Chapter Six : Embrace Humor for Happiness and Success

6. **It helps build trust.** You can build trust with the effective use of humor because humor often reveals the authentic person lurking under the professional mask. Numerous studies suggest that people who share a healthy, positive sense of humor tend to be more likeable and are reviewed as being more trustworthy. Humor is also viewed as a sign of intelligence. All of these characteristics, as well as the fact that humor is a fabulous icebreaker and can tear down walls, can help people build relationships in the workplace, and especially these days, relationships are critical to success.

7. **Humor can allow your company to stand out.** It can help companies stand out and go beyond with their customer service, garnering them a huge loyal following. If you want to stand out from the pack, using humor with your service is an effective way to do that.

8. **It can increase productivity.** Humor creates an upbeat atmosphere that encourages interaction, brainstorming of new ideas, and a feeling that there are few risks in thinking outside the box. All that leads to greater productivity. It also stands to reason that if you're in a more jovial atmosphere, you'll have more passion for what you do. Your work ethic will increase, and your enthusiasm will likely be contagious. It's a win-win for you and your company or business.

Michael Kerr was right when he said, "Humor is a connector, a builder, a catalyst. Humor doesn't just have the potential to make us financially richer, humor makes our lives richer." If you have read this chapter so far, it's time for you to embrace humor and use its techniques in your daily activities of daily living.

Humor and Smile Lead to Happiness and Success

A smile does magically and infectiously affect and please the people that you pass in the street, the person who serves you coffee, who opens the door for you, who interviews you for a job, and the people you share an elevator with. A smile's effect is not only contagious and powerful, but also can turn your world around and unlock opportunities.

Smiles have the power to break down the cold wall of indifference and a lonely heart that's blue. Given the reality that our enjoyment of life depends largely on how we manage and connect with people, a sincere smile is always the best strategy to build and establish rapport. A smile maintains attention, helps bolster open body language, and reassures the other person of your sincerity.

A smile is a powerful tool for peace. It's a natural, powerful gift that maintains peace through the expression of humility, warm welcome, understanding and love. It can hold together a nation and a peaceful world. The international bestselling author and activist Bryant H. McGill once said, "The greatest self is a peaceful smile, that always sees the world smiling back."

Research has shown that smiling releases serotonin—a neurotransmitter that produces feelings of happiness and wellbeing. When you want to tap into superpower and help yourself and others look great and competent, live longer, healthier, and happier lives— just smile.

The positivity that emanates from relying on the smile to guide our way helps us to treat others with kindness and compassion, realizing that all beings matter and that smooth running systems make life easier. Like our wilting potted plants that deserve watering, and the people we meet everywhere deserve our warmth.

In his famous book, *How To Win Friends and Influence People*, Dale Carnegie devoted an entire chapter on smiling. All what he said several decades ago is today supported by scientific evidence that shows that smiling is truly powerful. The good news, there are no language

Chapter Six : Embrace Humor for Happiness and Success

barriers when you smile. When the smile is on your face, everyone understands that your heart is at home.

Research has shown that people who smile regularly appear more confident, competent, and friendly. Try putting on a smile at meetings and business appointments. You might find people react to you differently.

In a study by the American Academy of Cosmetic Dentistry, participants were shown pictures of eight individuals and asked to quickly judge the people as to how attractive, happy, successful in their careers, friendly, interesting, kind, wealthy, popular with the opposite sex and sensitive to other people they were.

Two sets of photos were created, with each set showing four individuals before undergoing cosmetic dentistry and four after treatment. Two had mild improvements through cosmetic dentistry, two had moderate improvements and four had major improvements to their smiles. Respondents were not told that they were looking at dentistry but were asked to rate each person for the 10 characteristics.

The results indicated that an attractive smile does have a broad range of benefits. After comparing their rating after cosmetic dentistry to the ratings of the *before photos*, it was evident that the change was almost dramatic in the categories of attractive, popular, with the opposite sex, wealthy and successful in their careers. However, the change was also significant in all other areas. This means that those with an improved smile after cosmetic dentistry were also perceived to be more interesting, intelligent, sensitive, kind, and friendly.

This evidence supports a theory known as *halo effect* or, *what is beautiful is good* stenotype. When someone is attractive, they are assigned many other positive attributes that have nothing to do with looks. Therefore, someone with an attractive smile is often perceived to hold other positive traits.

It's a common belief that straight teeth and an appealing smile help us succeed in many avenues of life—whether it be in business or attracting the opposite sex. No wonder that the demand for cosmetic dentistry has risen. Teeth whitening, for example, has increased by more than 30 percent over the last decade.

I hope that what you have covered on humor is so inspiring that you won't again underestimate humor's potential to transform work and life. If you cultivate levity, it will make you and everyone around you more motivated, nimble, and effective at getting people to do what you want done. So, move and look closely for the sparks of levity in the nooks and crannies of your everyday experience (I promise they're there). And when you see these small sparks, give them oxygen, fan them into flames, play along, and build on them. I truly believe you can because by now the wheels of your life are already oiled by humor.

Now imagine if everyone in the world had this humor and levity mindset. Imagine if everyone searched for these sparks and spent more time walking through life on the precipice of a smile. Imagine that world! Now move and create it.

Do you want to cultivate a sense of humor in your life? The following section is going to teach how.

How to Develop Your Sense of Humor

In medicine, engineering, theology, or any other specialized discipline, students learn vocabulary, expressions, terminologies, and how to use tools of their chosen career. Similarly, I'm going to teach you humor techniques that you will use in the future to open opportunities for success.

Making it a habit to read articles, topics and books written humorously will greatly enhance your fluency because a person is what he or she reads. This is your starting point in your journey to become an interesting person. Learning the art of being a funny or interesting person is a must do if you want to make your life much more enjoyable and successful. For some people this comes easily and naturally, and for others, we might have to work a little harder to unlock it.

We don't all start by being the class clown or the joker. That's why the following tips were searched, tested, and proven to be effective humor techniques.

Watch More Stand-Up Comedies

This is as simple as it gets. To increase your sense of humor, watch more comedies. When you immerse yourself in a particular topic, you get good at it fast. You learn more effectively when you get involved in something enthusiastically. Similarly, you can refine your sense of humor by getting deeply interested in it. Watching stand-up comedies and following the jokes can have you rolling out of your seat in no time.

The law of attraction will help you increase your sense of humor by filtering out jokes, pickup lines and other metaphors that make people laugh.

Try To See the Funny Side to Almost Everything

If you really want to develop your sense of humor, then try to take something ordinary and make a joke out of it. There is a hidden joke behind every little event and situation you come across. Many comedians focus on the world around them to find comedic material. Others look to their past experiences, such as their childhood, or past relationships as a way to make people laugh.

Try making a goal of noticing funny things per day that happen to you. Through this technique, you'll begin to see humor in ordinary situations that everyone will appreciate. Try to find inspiration and material in the absurd and strange aspects of everyday life. What do you see strange in popular music, fashion, the holidays, current events, and the world around you? There are a lot of humor tools over there for you to use.

Learn Some Very Simple Jokes

In the beginning, you don't have to be secretive. Just go out and do some research! Try searching for stuff that you like and add funny, joke, or comedy to the end of your search. You'll find millions of things to make you laugh. Before telling your jokes, read the crowd. It's important to understand your audience. The jokes you'll share with your guy friends while out for drinks might be a little bit more sexual and explicit. Compare that to what you'll share with your relatives over dinner, which will be a bit wittier and conservative.

Get Comfortable with Yourself and Your Opinions About Life

Everyone has opinions about life, and in many cases, opinions can be humorous to other people. People who are naturally funny are typically willing to find humor in both themselves and their opinions. Think about opening up to others by sharing an embarrassing story about yourself. Be cautious, however, as self-deprecating jokes could make you or others feel uncomfortable.

If a story gets a good reaction, then keep telling that story. If not, shake it off and forget about it. Tick with something that is in good taste.

If Someone Doesn't Laugh, Don't Give Up

All comics will face criticism occasionally. The thing about jokes and your sense of humor you have to understand is that everyone won't always get it. In fact, there will probably be a moment where you finish a joke and hear crickets chirp. Don't make a big deal out of it. Shrug it off and move on.

Research Comedic Styles

Different comedic styles appeal to different people. Some people enjoy sarcastic and witty comments, others are good with jokes, some like impressions, and others still enjoy funny actions. All of these are legitimate methods of being funny, but it is best to pick something that fits your personality to be naturally funny. Keep trying and coming up with better materials to make your audience laugh, whether it is on a stage, or just among friends. Be clear when someone hurts your feelings with a joke and then forgive them and move on. Developing a sense of humor is much easier when you can forgive people.

Chapter Six: Embrace Humor for Happiness and Success

Become Humor Spotter

Look for humor around you, bumper stickers, blooper ads, funny cartoons, and amusing pictures. Being funny is a set of skills that can be learned and improved over time.

Keep A Funny File

Exceptionally funny people don't depend upon their memory to keep track of everything they discover that they find funny. In the old days, great comedians carried notebooks to jot down funny thoughts or observations and scrapbooks for news clippings that struck them as funny. Today, you can do that easily with your smartphone. If you have a funny thought, record it as an audio note. If you read a funny article, save the link in your bookmarks.

The world is a funny place and your existence within it probably is funnier. Accepting that fact is a blessing that gives you everything you need to see and craft stories daily. All you must do is document them and then tell someone.

Tell Stories

Use real-life stories. The beauty of using personal experiences as fodder for humor is that your life experience is unique, and stories based on it are original. A joke is a fake story that sets up for a punchline. If the punch line falls flat, you end up looking like a fool. Rather than tell jokes, exceptionally funny people tell relevant stories that have humorous elements. If people don't find a story funny, no big deal, because the story has a point beyond just being funny. If people laugh, then all the better.

Minimize Your Words

Brevity is levity. Comedians are forced to get to the funny part as quickly as possible. Identify the key part of your story and get there quickly. Cut all unnecessary elements. When it comes to the time you spend processing your thoughts may be a missed opportunity.

Hypothetically drop the mike like a comedian and end the show while everyone's still laughing.

Delay Funny

Put the funny part at the end of the sentence. For example, if a snake is the surprise or twist in your story, don't say, "There was a snake in the box." Say "In that box was a snake." That way, you're not still talking when the audience is meant to be laughing. This also makes your timing look awesome.

Use Callback

Callback brings together everything in the end. This is where you go back (callback) and reference items that just got a laugh and weave in something from items mentioned earlier in the conversation. This can be one of your jokes that worked or something funny or memorable from someone else. Remember, you don't have to tell a joke to be funny!

Visit A Naturally Funny Friend or Acquaintance

We all have friends who are always good for a laugh. What is it that makes them funny? When you see them, pay careful attention to what makes them funny. Is it their tone of voice, body language, content, general demeanor, or something else that makes them naturally funny? Identifying what it is that makes them funny will provide clues for how you can be naturally funny as well. Make a habit of spending more time around funny people and offer to share a funny story or joke of your own. Don't be afraid to contribute. Every little laugh counts. In fact, just a couple of genuine laughs a day will not only enhance your quality of life, improve your perspective, but also will surely rub off on you.

Include Laughter in Your Morning Routine

Many of us have a routine that we follow every morning to help set us up to have a great day. How about adding laughter to your morning routine? One way you can do this is by getting a calendar of jokes that will give you a quick laugh when you glance at the jokes for the day. This calendar that tickles your fancy should be put right next to your dressing mirror. Another idea is to get yourself a joke book and read one joke every morning. When you make it a habit, it will help reduce your stress, improve your mood, and boost your health and well-being.

Laugh More

Set the intent to laugh more. Take time to gather funny stuff on good days that will be ready on any bad day. With that you will be able to laugh every day. Stock your humor in an easily accessible place so you'll have it in times of need. Make a resolution or set the intent of laughing heartily as often as you can. Setting a goal to laugh more is as important as setting the goals to get more exercise, eat healthier, and drink plenty of water. Tell yourself: 'I resolve to laugh more,' and:

- Read the funny pages
- Check out your bookstore's humor section
- Play with a pet
- Become a member of a comedy club
- Goof around with children
- Do something silly.

Avoid Memorizing and Re-Telling Old Jokes

Telling well recited jokes, such as knock-knock jokes or inappropriate jokes, will turn people off to your sense of humor. In addition, trying to tell a joke you heard on TV will appear rehearsed and unnatural. Stick with your own observations. So, what if you really can't find the funny? Believe it or not, it's possible to laugh without experiencing a funny event—and simulated laughter can be just as beneficial as the real thing. It can even make exercise more fun and productive.

To add simulated laughter into your own life, search for laugh yoga or laugh therapy groups. Or you can start simply by laughing at other people's jokes, even if you don't find them funny. Both you and the other person will feel good, it will draw you closer together, and who knows, it may even lead to some spontaneous laughter.

Work On Your Timing When Telling A Story Or A Joke

Professional comedians say timing is everything and key to comic delivery. Stories and jokes are made more fun when the teller pauses right before the punchline to build drama and anticipation. You can also wait to laugh until a couple of seconds after the punchline, that way people can never be sure if you are joking or not. Always give your audience time to laugh before moving on to a difficult topic.

Keep stories short and simple, as too much background or too many tangents will distract the audience. Do not wait too long, seize the moment!

Make Jokes at Your Own Expense

Audiences appreciate when you make yourself the target of comedy. Don't laugh at others, laugh with others. Laughing with others brings people together and pokes fun at our common challenges. It will help them open- up and they will find it easier to laugh at both you and them. As a result, people will begin laughing and social anxiety will be reduced.

If you are with someone who can laugh at themselves, you can gently poke fun at them after you have done the same to yourself. Make sure you don't go too far, as this will turn a light-hearted situation into an awkward one.

Practice

Most of the time you can experiment with friends one on one to see how funny you are. The more you practice the more comfortable you will become. A good sense of humor doesn't emerge overnight.

Chapter Six : Embrace Humor for Happiness and Success

By starting small, you'll be on your way to being naturally funny in general conversations. The more you practice your jokes, your stories, and your timing, the funnier you will be.

Be Witty

If you know someone who takes being witty as seriously as you do, it might help to enlist them as a type of 'witty sparring partner.' If you are comfortable with it, you can also try your hand at wit in the real world (e.g., at dinner parties or family reunions). Part of this real world's exposure is in exposing yourself to the spontaneity that wit requires. You can polish your wit with a little knowledge of popular culture, words of a song or a good book.

Find a Little Kid You Can Hung Out With

Little kids haven't forgotten how to laugh yet. They'll laugh at just about anything, and there are few things more infectious than a little kid's laugh. Fundamentally, humor is about surprise. Young children laugh at the word 'underpants or poop.' It's because it's such a naughty surprise to see a book throw that word at them. Those two words are supposed to be hidden. If you talk to your little kid friend about those two words, you'll laugh a lot together.

Learn to Laugh at Yourself

If you can learn to laugh at yourself, you'll never be short of humorous material. Conan O'Brien is an example of how to make fun of yourself. Conan frequently makes fun of his own hair, his paleness and even his jokes that flop. Tell funny deprecating stories about yourself. Self-deprecating humor is one of the most attractive kinds of humor.

Take Up Something New

When you start something new—whether it's drawing, or performing a karate kick—your initial attempt will likely be clumsy and even ridiculous. That's funny. And since in the point above you learned how to laugh at yourself, taking up something new is very likely to result in lots of laughs.

Invite a few unmarried friends for coffee, and then tell them 'Take my wife or take my husband, please!' It sounds funny, doesn't it? What do you expect to come after 'Take my wife or husband'? Lots of laughter.

Do More of What Makes You Laugh

When was the last time you had a good laugh? What were you doing? Do more of that. If you think it's entertaining, tell it to others as well because you'll deliver the joke or story with so much excitement and enthusiasm.

Read A Funny Book

A genuine funny book is one of life's greatest pleasures and a garden of humor.

CHAPTER SEVEN

Practicing Gratitude Makes Our Lives Richer

Gratitude is an expression of being grateful and appreciative. It entails embracing what is good in things, experiences, and people. When you're thankful, you appreciate what you have and consider how it enriches your life. Think of gratitude or positive thinking as a seed. The more attention you pay to the good in your life—what you already have—the more it will grow and flourish. As a seed develops, it can turn into a source of nourishment, like a fruit or a vegetable, or something of beauty and admiration, like a flower. A warm-hearted seed of gratitude can also grow within an individual, transforming him or her into a larger than life, inspirational, and treasured human being.

Two other things are equally true with a seed. First, consider what happens if you neglect the seed. It will stop growing, choke, and die. You will not profit from its potential, nor will anyone else.

Second, think carefully about the seed you have selected. If you plant the wrong seed and nourish it, it becomes a weed, hindering not only your personal growth but that of others. Eventually, it will grow uncontrollably, leaving ugliness and misery in the wake. By then, you may be near the end of your life, filled with regret, wallowing in disappointment, and entangled within a web of negative thoughts.

As you can tell from the above, positive thinking focuses on the positive aspect of life. Positive thinking, in fact, is remarkably easy to practice since everyone has something to be grateful for—be it family, a promotion, good health, shelter, and so on. Before we learn how to practice it, let us see its purpose in life.

The Purpose of Gratitude

People can use gratitude to form new social relations or to strengthen current ones. Acts of gratitude can be used to apologize, make amends, and help solve other problems.

Alternatively, people may feel gracious because it can be an intrinsically rewarding process. Simply being grateful for being alive is a great way to motivate oneself to seize the day. The idea that tomorrow is not guaranteed is a strong motivator for some people to be their "best self" today.

It takes vigilance to cultivate an attitude of gratitude because most of us are culturally conditioned to focus on what we don't have rather than what we do have. Sometimes we focus so much on the difficulties and challenges of our climb that we lose sight of being grateful for having that mountain to climb.

Appreciation and gratitude for the big and small things in life are often overlooked, and yet we have so much to be grateful for. If you have a roof over your head, a warm bed, food in your fridge, and clothes and shoes in your closet, you're better off than 74 percent of the world's population as it stands now. Hard to believe, but it's true. If you eat three meals a day, you're better off than one billion people on Earth who have access to one meal a day or none.

Lately there has been a lot of talk about gratitude, especially on social media. But talking about gratitude and practicing it are two different things. Practicing it means proactively seeking reasons to be grateful and then expressing appreciation.

How to Practice Gratitude

Becoming a more grateful individual is a lifelong pursuit. You aren't likely to instantly change how you are hardwired to view the world. Those pessimistic thoughts that run through your mind when the car in front of you cuts you off won't go away. But you can train your brain to become more aware of the positive around you.

With the simple act of acknowledging a few things you are grateful for, you become more open to recognizing these moments as they happen throughout the day. Becoming more grateful means shifting your mindset to one that embraces positivity.

Maintain a Gratitude Journal

Journaling is one of the most therapeutic activities we can engage in. When you write down your thoughts, you can gain perspective and see more clearly where you are coming from and where you are going. A gratitude journal helps you zero in on the things you should be grateful for in your life. A few things to keep in mind with your gratitude journal are:

1. **Go for Depth.** There is no need to keep a journal if you will be doing so superficially. You need to go beyond just listing the things you think you should be grateful for; you need to dig deep and think about *why* those things are important to you. Elaborate, don't just jot down bullet points. For example, a friend may have visited you at home. Instead of just noting the visit, reflect on the last time you saw each other, what you did during the visit, what your friend's visit meant to you, and whether you conveyed you were thankful to your friend for their visit.

2. **Get Personal.** While being grateful for the things you have in your life is great, you should get personal and talk more about the people you should be grateful for and grateful to.

   For example, when you receive a gift, instead of just saying to others "I got such-and-such," elaborate on who gave you the gift, the atmosphere at that time, how you felt when you received it, and what purpose the person's gift will serve. In other words, do not focus on the gift, focus more on the gift-giver.

3. **Try Subtraction.** A good way to determine what you are grateful for is to use the subtraction method. With this method, you think about how your life would be if you didn't have specific people and things in your life. First, think of your eyesight and what it would mean if you could not see. Blindfold yourself for a minute or two and try to complete your usual chores. This will help you get a feel for what it would be like to lose your vision. You should feel immensely grateful for being able to see.

   For another experiment, consider what your life would be like without peace in your country. Think of a distant war-torn region. Read a story or two on life there amidst strife, conflict, and destruction. Imagine being there with your loved ones. Next, turn your thoughts back to your real life. Again, you cannot help but feel thankful. Peace is something many people enjoy yet never feel it is worth being thankful for.

Record Unexpected Events.

Sometimes people surprise you. What surprises you might not be a big thing; it could be a simple gesture. Maybe a neighbor unexpectedly dropped by to invite you to dinner. Or maybe a colleague said a nice word about you to another person. Maybe a child smiled at you for no reason. You should take note of such surprises because they will remind you that life is worth living and that there is much to be grateful for.

Even though a kind gesture or word may appear insignificant, you should allow yourself a moment to appreciate it.

Do Not Overdo It.

When it comes to writing down the things you are grateful for, do not overdo it. Instead of having a long list, limit the list of things you are grateful for to five and elaborate on those things and your feelings about them. It would also help if you occasionally read your journal (perhaps weekly or bi-weekly). This will remind you of the positive things happening in your life.

Write a Thank You Note

You can make yourself happier and nurture your relationship with another person by writing a thank-you letter or email expressing your enjoyment and appreciation of the person's impact on your life. Send it, or better yet, deliver and read it in person if possible. Make a habit of sending at least one gratitude letter a month. Occasionally, write one to yourself.

Thank Someone Mentally

It may help just to think about someone who has done something nice for you, and mentally thank the individual. This can be done by saying in your heart the following: I'm so grateful, I appreciate it, I couldn't have done it without you, or thanks for having my back.

Pray

People who are religious or believe in a higher power can use prayer to cultivate gratitude. Muslims demonstrate gratitude during the five daily prayers. Considering the extent of our blessings, we should be demonstrating gratitude even more than five times a day.

Meditate

Mindfulness meditation involves focusing on the present without judgement. Although people often focus on a word or phrase (such as "peace"), it's also possible to focus on what you're grateful for (the warmth of the sun, a pleasant sound, and so on).

Being grateful is much more important than most average people realize. Indeed, many successful individuals claim that they are where they are now due to practicing gratitude. In *The Science of Getting Rich*, Wallace Wattles writes, "The grateful mind is constantly fixed upon the best. Therefore, it tends to become the best; it takes the form or character of the best and will receive the best."

The question is: Can it create what wasn't there before? Tangible things like an opportunity, or a great space to live in, or actual personal wealth? The answer is a big yes.

Gratitude Is the Key to Unlocking Happiness and Success

We've been thinking and doing things backwards. Success doesn't lead to gratitude and happiness. *Success starts with gratitude.* If you want to be successful, start with gratitude! Gratitude leads to increased happiness, which leads to motivation to achieve your goals. Research has demonstrated many times over the many benefits of practicing gratitude. Most importantly, gratitude leads to increased levels of happiness. Increased levels of happiness lead to more motivation and drive to achieve your goals. Achieving goals in turn leads to increased levels of happiness.

Once you enter this cycle of feeling happy, succeeding at your goals, and in turn feeding back into your happiness levels, life is pretty good. It's easy to feel appreciative for what you have and the progress that you have made. If you have trouble entering this feedback loop of happiness and goal success, try starting with gratitude first. You can't just tell yourself to be happier. However, you can take time out of your day to reflect on the things in your life that you are grateful for.

Happiness and Gratitude Increase Goal Success

When you feel happy, you feel optimistic and energized. This motivated energy leads to action. And action is the vital ingredient to goal success. If you think back to the time you were most successful at accomplishing your goals, what was the driving force behind your actions? Often it's a reason that is incredibly important to you. But no matter how big the *why* behind the goal, if you feel depressed and unmotivated, you probably won't get very far. If we lead with happiness, then we can finally find success.

As we make progress on our goals, we feel more confident, accomplished, and motivated. These positive emotions fuel our progress even further. The happier we feel, the more progress we make. While this positive feedback loop won't spiral out of control as you become increasingly manic, it can fuel success. Research even demonstrates that small successes motivate you to achieve larger successes.

Now that we know how happiness and gratitude lead to success, it's time to learn all the benefits of positive thinking.

Why Being Grateful Is Important

Gratitude offers numerous benefits once you start practicing it. Some of these benefits are:

1. Enhanced Well-Being

Expressing your thanks can improve your overall sense of well-being. Grateful people are more agreeable, more open, and less neurotic. Furthermore, gratitude is related inversely to depression, and positively to life satisfaction. This is not to say that "depressed people" should simply be more grateful, as depression is a very complicated disease. Instead, perhaps gratitude practices need to be a part of the therapy and treatment for people who struggle with depression.

2. Deeper Relationships

Gratitude is also a powerful tool for strengthening interpersonal relationships. People who express their gratitude for each other tend to be more willing to forgive others and less narcissistic. Giving thanks to those who have helped you strengthen your relationships and who promote relationships formation and maintenance, as well as relationship connection and satisfaction, is a true act of gratitude.

3. Improved Optimism

Gratitude is the antidote for the toxic things that come into our lives. Simply put, gratitude fosters optimism, which strengthens hope. That's why it's hard to imagine more effective soul medicine than gratitude.

4. Increased Happiness

Steven M. Toepfer, Kelly Cichy, and Patti Petters conducted a study in 2012 asking people to write and deliver a letter to someone for whom they were grateful. After the task, their happiness levels and life satisfaction were dramatically impacted—even a week later.

In the pursuit of happiness and life satisfaction, gratitude offers a long-lasting effect in a positive-feedback loop of sorts. Thus, the more gratitude we experience and express, the more situations and people we may find to express gratitude towards.

5. Stronger Self-Control

Self-control helps with discipline and focus. Our long-term well-being can benefit from self-control, for example, when someone who is trying to quit smoking resists cigarettes. Self-control helps us stick to the "better choice" for our long-term health, financial future, and well-being.

A study by DeStefano and others in 2014 found that self-control significantly increased when subjects chose gratitude. One of the study's authors, Professor Ye Li, said: "Showing that emotion can foster self-control and discovering a way to reduce impatience with a simple gratitude exercise opens up tremendous possibilities for reducing a wide range of societal ills from impulse buying and insufficient savings to obesity and smoking."

Being thankful can provide us with the resolve we need to make choices in our lives that serve us emotionally and physically in the long run. There are so many applications to using gratitude as a path towards healthier humans and communities. You can google them for more details.

6. Better Physical and Mental Health

Research performed in 2015 found that patients with heart failure who completed gratitude journals showed reduced inflammation, improved sleep, and better moods; this reduced their symptoms of heart failure after only eight weeks.

The link between the mind and the body aligns with how gratitude can have a double benefit. For example, the feeling of appreciation helps us to have healthier minds, and with that healthier bodies.

7. An Overall Better Life

Over the last two decades, the evidence supporting the benefits of gratitude has increased a lot. Adults who feel grateful have more energy, more optimism, more social connections, and more happiness than those who do not, according to studies conducted over the past decade. They're also less likely to be depressed, envious, greedy, or alcoholics.

8. Stronger Athleticism

Studies from researcher Lung Hung Chen of Taiwan Sports University found that an athlete's level of gratitude for their success can influence their levels of well-being. More specifically, adolescent athletes who are more grateful in life are also more satisfied and tend to have higher levels of self-esteem.

Gratitude also affects sports fans. Fans' levels of gratitude influence their happiness, connection, and how they identify with a team. In turn, stronger fan support and pride can influence the performance and pride of the players themselves for representing a greater team.

Teri McKeever has applied these findings to her team, and with incredible success. As the women's swimming and diving coach at the University of California at Berkeley, McKeever incorporated gratitude exercises into her team practices—and won three NCAA National Championships in her twenty-year career there.

9. Stronger Neurologically Based Morality

Neuroscience is beginning to explore what gratitude does to the mysterious human brain. One study conducted by Glenn R. Fox and Jonas Kaplan of the University of Southern California measured the brain's response to feelings of gratitude with functional magnetic resonance imaging (MRI). These researchers elicited feelings of gratitude from their participants and found that gratitude increased activity in areas of the brain that deal with morality, rewards, and judgement.

10. Gratitude Enhances Empathy

Gratitude enhances your empathy by realigning your perspective, allowing you to appreciate the little things in your life and understand others' difficulties. Think of it this way: When you fail to feel thankful for what you have, you will find it difficult to understand how others' lack of those very things affects them. However, when you start thinking about the things you should be grateful for, you'll understand that others may not have such perfect lives. This will change how you relate to them. When this happens, you will be more understanding and less aggressive and judgmental when dealing with others.

11. Gratitude Helps Deal with Hardships

A study at Eastern Washington University explored the link between gratefulness and dealing with difficult experiences. Participants were asked to recall and report on an unpleasant emotional impact. Those who thought about the positive aspects generally responded more positively than those who thought only about the memory in general terms. The study found that those with gratitude showed more memory closure, less unpleasant emotional impact, and less intrusiveness of the open memory than others.

12. Gratitude Can Improve Your Sleep

There is also evidence that gratitude can improve your sleep quality. Those who are struggling with their sleep will know how difficult it can make life, so any practice that can improve your sleep will be welcome.

The things that keep most of us up at night are things that aren't going well in our lives. Instead of having a restful sleep, we fret about bills that need to be paid, conflicts at work, family troubles, or things we want to own. Stressed out and agitated, we lie awake for hours on end. We then start the next day exhausted and in low spirits.

The experts tell us that stress relief holds the key to curing insomnia. Such relief can take many forms, including exercise, time off from work, and counseling. One often overlooked way to reduce stress is to stop dwelling on all the things going wrong, and instead focus on everything that is going right. In other words, try positive thinking. This will put you in a relaxed, contended frame of mind. You'll sleep through the night knowing you have a lot to be thankful for.

13. Gratitude Can Reduce Preoccupation with Materialism

Materialism in society induces insatiable desires among individuals to want more wealth and consumer goods. Instead of allowing you to appreciate what you already have, it shifts your thoughts to the things you want but don't necessarily need.

On the other hand, positive thinking helps you see what is special and enjoyable about your life. Even the smallest things can seem like a precious gift when you adopt an attitude of gratitude. Several studies have suggested that practicing gratitude can also make you more satisfied with what you do for a living. All of these are positive traits for whatever you do, but evidence doesn't end there. A 2015 study highlighted that gratitude also helps people find meaning in their daily activities.

14. Gratitude Can Increase and Improve Your Chances of Success

Good news for those with a burning desire to succeed. Scientific research from notable psychologists shows that grateful people are more likely to be happy and successful. No wonder—gratitude makes you feel good about your accomplishments, which in turn motivates you to tackle other tasks geared towards helping you achieve more goals. Did you know that gratitude can enhance positive emotions? Research from 2017 found that positive emotions allow people to build psychological, intellectual, and social resources. What's more, practices such as gratitude may play a role in motivating individuals to engage in positive behaviors leading to self-improvement.

15. Improved Psychological Health

Toxic emotions mess up your psychological health. When you dwell on negative feelings, especially those concerning yourself, you fall into a state of despair. Darkness enshrouds your mind and dampens your spirit.

Gratitude removes you from that state. It shifts your focus from toxic thoughts to uplifting emotions. Thinking about what you are grateful for recalibrates your mind and brings about a brighter outlook. Happiness begins to flicker and then well up within your soul, shining light and overpowering the darkness in the world around you.

Conclusion

Practicing positive thinking is not always an easy task. Some days you will wonder why you are alive and why you should go on. Everyone has been there, and problems are a part of life.

Nevertheless, with a bit of effort practicing the strategies described in this chapter, a definite pattern will emerge over the next few days, weeks, and years. You will find it easier to see the good in life, in others, and, most importantly, in yourself. If, and when difficulties arise, you will persevere, appreciating what you have and who you are, learning from your experience, and facing the future with confidence.

Take care to plant and nurture seeds of gratitude in your mind and in your heart and you will harvest joy, happiness, and success. Try to find blessings in everything and in everyone. Adopt positive thinking as part of your life to improve yourself and make the world a better place.

CHAPTER EIGHT

Happiness Is the Key to Success

For untold generations, we have been led to believe that happiness orbited around success. That if we work hard enough, we will be successful, and only if we are successful will we become happy. Now, thanks to breakthroughs in the burgeoning field of positive psychology, we are learning that the opposite is true. When we are happy—when our mindset and mood are positive—we are smarter, more motivated, and thus more successful. Happiness is the center, and success revolves around it.

The most successful people, the ones with the competitive edge, don't look at happiness as some distant reward for their achievements; they are the ones who capitalize on the positive and reap the rewards at every turn.

The Science of Happiness

According to science, there is no single meaning; happiness is relative to the person experiencing it. Therefore, scientists often refer to it as "subjective well-being" because it's based on how we each feel about our own lives. In essence, the best judge of how happy you are is you. To empirically study happiness then, scientists must rely on individual self-reports. Thankfully, after years of testing and honing survey questions of people around the world, researchers have developed self-report metrics that accurately and reliably measure individual happiness.

So how do scientists define happiness? Essentially, as the experience of positive emotions—pleasure combined with deeper feelings of meaning and purpose. Happiness implies a positive mood in the present and a positive outlook for the future. Martin Seligman, the pioneer of positive psychology, has broken it down into three measurable components: pleasure, engagement, and meaning. His studies have confirmed that people who pursue only pleasure experience only part of the benefits happiness can bring, while those who pursue all three routes lead the fullest lives. Perhaps the most accurate term for happiness then is the one Aristotle used: *eudaimonia*, which translates not directly to "happiness" but to "human flourishing." This definition really resonates with me because it acknowledges that happiness is not all about yellow smiley faces and rainbows. For me, happiness is the joy we feel striving for our potential.

The chief engine of happiness is positive emotions, since happiness is, above all else, a feeling. Barbara Fredrickson, a researcher at the University of North Carolina and perhaps the world's leading expert on the subject, details the ten most positive emotions: "joy, gratitude, serenity, interest, hope, pride, amusement, inspiration, awe, and love." This paints a far richer picture of happiness than that ubiquitous yellow smiley face, which doesn't leave much room for nuance. But as we are about to see, happiness is even more than a feeling—it's also an indispensable ingredient of our success.

Happiness Leads to Success at Work

Hoping that some of the readers of *How to Succeed After 55* are still working, I want to demonstrate how happiness leads to success at work. Researchers brought together the results of over 200 scientific studies on nearly 275,000 people and found that happiness leads to success in nearly every domain of our lives, including marriage, health, friendship, community involvement, creativity, and our jobs, careers, and business. Data abounds showing that happy workers have higher levels of productivity, produce higher sales, perform better in leadership positions, and receive higher performance ratings and pay. They also enjoy more job security and are less likely to take sick days, to quit, or to become burned out. Happy CEOs are more likely to lead teams of employees who are both happy and healthy, and who find their work climate conducive to high performance. The list of the benefits of happiness in the workplace goes on and on.

Different Definitions of Happiness

In general, happiness is understood as the positive emotions we have regarding the pleasurable activities we take part in throughout our daily lives. As already mentioned above, pleasure, comfort, gratitude, hope, inspiration, and success are examples of positive emotions that increase our happiness and move us to flourish.

For example, if you can imagine the future being bright, it lifts your energy and gooses chemistry in your body that produces a sensation of happiness. I find it useful to daydream that the future will be better than today, by far. I like to imagine a future that is spectacular and breathtaking. The daydreams need not be accurate in terms of predicting the future. Simply imagining a better future hacks your brain chemistry and provides you with the sensation of happiness today. Being happy raises your energy level and makes it easier to pursue the steps towards real-world happiness.

The next important thing to remember about happiness is that it's not a mystery of the mind and it's not magic. Happiness is the natural state for most people whenever they feel healthy, have flexible schedules, and expect the future to be bright. The other elements of happiness can also include being famous, having a soulmate, achieving recognition, or a feeling of importance, and lots more.

Happiness means different things to different people.

- In her book, *The How of Happiness*, Sonja Lyubomirsky, a professor of psychology at the University of California, defines happiness as "the experience of joy, contentment, or positive well-being, combined with a sense that one's life is good, meaningful, and worthwhile."

- The Merriam-Webster dictionary defines happiness as: a state of well-being and contentment; a pleasurable or satisfying experience.

- Author Ayn Rand says: "Happiness is that state of consciousness which proceeds from the achievement of one's values."

- Mahatma Gandhi says: "Happiness is when what you think, what you say, and what you do are in harmony."

- To psychological researchers, the two components of subjective well-being are "feelings of happiness" and "thoughts of satisfaction with life."

Every individual has their own definition of what makes them happy. But extensive research on happiness has shown that there are certain needs that must be satisfied to achieve this emotional state. What I am referring to is long-term happiness and not the momentary feelings of joy we experience in our everyday lives.

There are four levels of happiness.

1. **Physical pleasure and immediate gratification.** This form of happiness is relatively short-lived and shallow.

2. **Passion.** Whether it's a hobby or getting recognition at your job, being passionate about something is an excellent source of happiness.

3. **Purpose.** When you feel like your talents and skills allow you to serve others and are part of something bigger, this can give you a sense of purpose, fulfillment and long-term happiness.

4. **Ultimate Good.** The fourth level of happiness is known as ultimate good. This is a fundamental desire we have as human beings for perfect truth, goodness, beauty, and love.

Five different dimensions of well-being:

1. **Positive emotions.** This can be pleasure caused by delicious food, a warm bed, anything that pleases one of the five senses.

2. **Engagement or Flow.** The experience of an enjoyable and challenging activity.

3. **Relationships.** Social ties are an extremely reliable factor of happiness.

4. **Meaning.** Belonging to something bigger than ourselves.

5. **Accomplishment.** The achievement of goals.

Varied Results and Views on the Cause of Happiness

Since the 1960s, scientific disciplines have conducted research on happiness, to determine how humans can live happier lives. The scientific pursuit of positive emotion and happiness is the pillar of positive psychology, first proposed in 1998 by Martin Seligman.

The studies have come up with varied results and views on the cause of happiness. Here are some of their findings:

- One result from the seventy-five-year Grant Study of Harvard undergraduates shows that loving relationships, especially with parents, have a great impact on our well-being in our later years.

- Based on twin studies, Sonja Lyubomirsky concludes that 50 percent of our happiness level is determined by our genes, 40 percent is related to our self-control, and 10 percent is influenced by personal situations and life circumstances.

- Finnish research on 701 individuals showed that happiness activates our whole body, from the head down to the legs.

- People can extract more pleasure out of ordinary experiences as they age. Younger people define their happiness more by extraordinary experiences.

- Excessive money, beyond what we need to feed, clothe, and house ourselves, only increases happiness by a fraction.

- A Harvard Business School study found that we are happier when we spend money on others, rather than on ourselves.

- Relationships are keys to long-term happiness. The effect is strongest in married couples, but deep, meaningful relationships with others have the same impact.

- Surveys by Gallup, the National Research Center, and the Pew organization state that people who are more spiritual tend to be happier than those who are not.

- Religious people who benefit from social contact and peer support also showed an increased tendency to be happy and satisfied with their lives.

- Research findings show that eight hugs a day can increase your levels of oxytocin, and result in a happier you. A higher level of oxytocin is attributed to feelings of trust and camaraderie.

- A 2008 study from the University of Bristol found that

people's moods significantly improve after engaging in exercise.

- Acts of kindness make people more well liked and accepted. This leads to social acceptance and an improved self-image. (University of British Columbia, 2012.)

- In a significant study by the University of California in 2008, researchers concluded that surrounding yourself with happy people will increase the possibility of your future happiness. Happiness is said to be contagious.

- The experience of being able to buy material things causes happiness, not the possession itself. It satisfies our higher-order needs for social connectedness and vitality and heightens the feeling of being alive. (San Francisco State University, 2009.)

Happiness Lifts Your Spirits

If happiness is a universal goal, then we need to understand its cause and effect. We need to know why it's so important to us. Why are we so hung up on being happy? The goal is simply to lift your spirits and put you in a more positive mindset, so you can reap all the benefits of being happy.

Meditation

Neuroscientists have found that monks who spend years meditating actually grow their left prefrontal cortex, the part of the brain most responsible for feeling happy. But don't worry, you don't have to spend years in sequestered, celibate silence to experience a boost. Take just five minutes each day to watch your breath go in and out. While you do so, try to remain patient. If you find your mind drifting, just slowly bring it back to focus. Meditation takes practice, but it's one of the most powerful happiness interventions. Studies have shown that in the minutes right after meditating, we experience feelings of calm and contentment, as well as heightened awareness and empathy. Research also shows that regular meditation can even permanently rewire the brain to raise levels of happiness, lower stress, and improve immune function.

Find Something to Look Forward To

One study found that people who thought that just watching their favorite movie raised their endorphin levels by 27 percent. Often the most enjoyable part of an activity is the anticipation. If you can't take the time for a vacation right now, or even a night out with friends, put something on the calendar—even if it's a month or a year down the road. Then wherever you need a boost of happiness, remind yourself about it. Anticipating future rewards can light up the pleasure centers in your brain as much as the actual reward will.

Commit Conscious Acts of Kindness

A long line of empirical research, including one study of 2,000 people, has shown that acts of altruism—giving to friends and strangers alike—decrease stress and strongly contribute to enhanced mental health. Sonja Lyubomirsky, a leading researcher and author of *The How of Happiness*, has found that individuals told to complete five acts of kindness over the course of a day report feeling much happier than control groups and that the feeling lasts for many subsequent days far after the exercise is over. To try this yourself, pick one day a week and make a point of committing five acts of kindness. But if you want to reap the psychological benefit, make sure you do these things deliberately and consciously—you can't just look back over the last twenty-four hours and declare your acts post hoc. ("Oh yeah, I held the door for that guy coming out of the bank. That was nice.") And they need not be grand gestures either. One of my favorite acts is to donate to Covenant House serving youth who are homeless in Toronto.

Infuse Positivity into Your Surroundings

While we may not always have complete control over our surroundings, we can make specific efforts to infuse them with positivity. Think about your office: What feelings does it inspire? People who flank their computers with pictures of loved ones aren't just decorating—they're ensuring a hit of positive emotions each time they glance in that direction. Making time to go outside on a nice day also delivers a huge advantage; one study found that spending twenty minutes outside in good weather not only boosted the mood, but broadened thinking and improved working memory.

Exercise

You have probably heard that exercise releases pleasure-inducing chemicals called endorphins, but that is not its only benefit. Physical activity can boost our mood and enhance our work performance in a number of other ways as well, by improving motivation and feelings of mastery, reducing stress and anxiety, and helping us get into flow—that "locked in" feeling of total engagement that we usually get when we're at our most productive.

Spend Money, but Not on Stuff

Contrary to the popular saying, money can buy happiness, but only if used to do things as opposed to simply having things. In his book *Luxury Fever*, Robert Frank explains that while the positive feelings we get from material objects are frustratingly fleeting, spending money on experiences, especially ones with other people, produces positive emotions that are both more meaningful and more lasting. For instance, when researchers interviewed more than 150 people about their recent purchases, they found that money spent on activities—such as concerts and group dinners out—brought far more pleasure than material purchases like shoes, televisions, or expensive watches. Spending money on others, called "prosocial spending," also boosts happiness.

Exercise a Signature Strength

Everyone is good at something—perhaps you give excellent advice, or you're great with kids, or you whip up a mean batch of blueberry pancakes. Each time we use a skill, whatever it is, we experience a burst of positivity. If you find yourself in need of a happiness booster, revisit a talent you haven't used in a while.

Even more fulfilling than using a skill, though, is exercising a strength of character, a trait that is deeply embedded in who we are. A team of psychologists recently catalogued the twenty-four cross-cultural character strengths that most contribute to human flourishing. They then developed a comprehensive survey that identifies an individual's top-five, or "signature," strengths. When 577 volunteers were encouraged to pick one of their signature strengths and use it in a new way each day for a week, they became significantly happier and less depressed than those in the control groups. And these benefits lasted: Even after the experiment was over their levels of happiness remained heightened a full six months later.

The same team of psychologists found that the more you use your signature strengths, the happier you become. One of mine is the "love of learning," and I feel noticeably depleted on the days I don't use this strength. So, I find opportunities to incorporate learning into my boring daily tasks.

As you integrate these happiness exercises into your life, you'll not only start to feel better, but you'll also start to notice how your enhanced positivity makes you more efficient, motivated, and productive, and opens opportunities for greater achievement. But the happiness doesn't end there. By changing how you work, and the way you lead the people around you, you can enhance the success of your team and your whole organization or business.

It's time to move from how happiness leads to the success of individuals, organizations, and businesses and explore its influence on global organizations and nations around the world.

Chapter Eight : Happiness Is the Key to Success

The Global Pursuit of Happiness

In world economic circles, Professor Richard Easterlin investigated the relationship between money and well-being. The Easterlin paradox, "money doesn't buy happiness," sparked a new wave of thinking about wealth and well-being, or happiness.

This new wave started in the Kingdom of Bhutan. In 1972, Bhutan declared, "Gross National Happiness is more important than Gross Domestic Product." They chose to pursue a policy of happiness rather than a focus on economic growth tracked via their gross domestic product (GDP). Since then, Bhutan has been both ranked the happiest country in Asia, and the ninety-fifth happiest country in the world, according to the 2021 World Happiness Report. It also has one of the fastest growing economies in Asia. Based on what the Kingdom of Bhutan has taught the world, happiness leads to greater success in life.

More global organizations and nations are becoming aware and supportive of the importance of happiness in today's world. This has led to the United Nations inviting nations to take part in a happiness survey, resulting in the "World Happiness Report," a basis for which to steer public policy.

On June 28, 2012, the United Nations also established World Happiness Day, which is observed on March 20. It was established because of Bhutan's efforts and their Gross National Happiness Initiative.

Ruut Veenhoven, a world authority on the scientific study of happiness in the sense of subjective enjoyment of life, was one of the sources of inspiration for the United Nations adopting happiness measures. Veenhoven is a South African of Dutch origin, and a founding member of the World Database of Happiness, which is a comprehensive scientific repository of happiness measures worldwide. The objective of this organization is to provide a coordinated collection of data, with common interpretation according to a scientifically validated happiness theory, model, and body of research.

Measures of Happiness

At this point, you might be wondering: Is it possible to measure happiness? Many psychologists have devoted their careers to answering this question, and in short, the answer is yes.

Happiness can be measured by these three factors:

- The presence of positive emotions.
- The absence of negative emotions, and
- Life satisfaction.

It is a uniquely subjective experience, which means that nobody is better at reporting on someone's happiness than the individuals themselves. For this reason, scales, self-reporting measures, and questionnaires are the most common formats for measuring happiness. The most recognized examples are the following:

1. **The PANAS (Positive Affect and Negative Affect Schedule).** The PANAS is a self-report questionnaire that consists of two ten item scales to measure both positive and negative effects. Each item is rated on a five-point scale from 1 (not at all) to 5 (very much). The measure has been used mainly as a research tool in group studies but can be utilized within clinical and non-clinical populations as well.

2. **The SWLS (Satisfaction with Life Scale).** This scale was developed to assess satisfaction with people's lives. The scale does not assess satisfaction with specific domains, such as health or finances, but allows subjects to integrate and weigh these domains in whatever way they choose. It takes a few minutes to complete.

3. **The SHS (Subjective Happiness Scale).** This is a four item self-report measure developed to assess an individual's overall happiness as measured through self-evaluation.

Chapter Eight : Happiness Is the Key to Success

The response format is a seven- point Likert-type scale questionnaire. A single composite score is computed by averaging the responses to the four items following reverse coding of the fourth item. Scores range from 1.0 to 7.0, with higher scores reflecting greater happiness.

There are many other instruments available to measure happiness that have been proven reliable and valid over time.

As already mentioned repeatedly above, happiness creates success everywhere. Success is not the key to happiness. Happiness is the key to success. If you love what you're doing, you will be successful. Success is your definition of a goal. If you think about your death, wake, and funeral, you can better understand your idea of success. What would people say about you? If you carefully consider what you want to be said at your funeral, you will find your definition of success.

Richard Branson, founder of the Virgin Group, believes success is engagement. American author Maya Angelou believes success is enjoying your work, and Zappos CEO Tony Hsieh says success is living in line with your values. These definitions of three individuals support the science of happiness that says there is no single definition of happiness or success.

CHAPTER NINE

Brain Health Is Central to All Health and Success

When your brain works right, you are happier, healthier, and it makes you wealthier (because you make better decisions) and more successful in everything you do.

Seriously, you are in a war for the health of your brain. Just about everywhere you go, you are offered toxic food that will kill you early. Be aware that some weapons of mass destruction of your brain are processed, pesticide-sprayed, high-glycemic, low-fiber foods. Such fare is destroying the health of people all over the world. Two-thirds of us are overweight or obese, 50 percent are diabetic or prediabetic, and 60 percent are hypertensive—all conditions that damage the brain.

You Must Become a Brain Warrior

In this chapter, I will tell you how to become a brain warrior and a memory rescuer too. That's because one of the most important symptoms of an unhealthy brain are memory problems. Once your memory starts to slip, everything in your life such as health, relationships, work, and finances, becomes more difficult to manage. Such problems can even strip you of your independence. Let me be clear: I love my children very much, but I never want to live with them. I never want to be a burden to them, and I would prefer they not make decisions for me. I don't want them deciding what I will wear and eat. If this is true for you, too, you need to think about your brain now, not twenty years from now. The truly exciting news is that you can start to change your brain and memory, beginning today. Join me on a fascinating and important journey into improving your brain memory and your life.

Memory Is Life

Our memories are such a part of us that we often take them for granted. Yet when our memory is damaged, the costs can be high. A diminished memory can rob us of our ability to make good decisions and disconnect us from those we love. Memory problems limit our success at work and in business, steal our independence, and ultimately make us vulnerable to anyone who might take advantage of us.

Yet new research suggests that a "memory rescue" program, like the one presented in this chapter, can dramatically improve memory, and can prevent and sometimes even reverse some forms of dementia. Given how most doctors approach this issue, however, you cannot count on traditional medicine to rescue your memory.

The Memory Rescue Promise

Memory Rescue will teach you the most common reasons for memory loss and help you identify the specific factors affecting your brain health. It will then provide you with a step-by-step approach to get your memory back, strengthen it, and keep it healthy for a lifetime.

Chapter Nine: Brain Health Is Central to All Health and Success

You will learn:

- How to assess your brain on a regular basis to identify issues early.
- How to test for each risk factor.
- Strategies to decrease or eliminate avoidable risks through exercises, nutritional supplementation, and diet.
- How to follow the Memory Rescue Diet (one of the most powerful weapons for memory sustainability)
- Memory training and workouts to keep your brain sharp
- Innovative strategies to enhance brain function

Before we dive into those details, join me on a fascinating and important journey into your brain, the place where memories are truly made. If you have trouble remembering things, memory loss is no laughing matter. If you often have no idea where you put your keys and sometimes find them in the refrigerator next to the yogurt, that's not normal. If any of this sounds familiar, it's time for you to love your brain because it runs everything in your life. It makes you who you are, producing your thoughts, feelings, plans, and behaviors. It's the organ that enables you to learn, love, and work, and it is at the center of every decision you make. A healthy brain leads to better decision making, which in turn leads to better relationships, job performance, finances, physical health, and overall happiness.

Even though your brain makes up only about 2 percent of your body's weight (about three pounds), it uses 20 to 30 percent of the calories you take in, as well as 20 percent of the oxygen and blood flow in your body. To strengthen your memory, it's important to understand how a healthy brain works and the role each of the four regions plays in the creation, storage, and retrieval of memories. Get ready for a fascinating tour of the brain. My goal as your guide is for you to come away with a sense of wonder, awe, and a better grasp of why it's so important to love your brain. You get only one and taking care of your unique brain will contribute to your living a happier, healthier, more memorable life.

The Brain Is Divided into Four Regions

The brain's main regions or lobes are:

- Frontal lobes and prefrontal cortex
- Temporal lobes
- Parietal lobes
- Occipital lobes

The front lobes are divided into three sections: the motor cortex, which controls the body's motor movements such as jumping, chewing, and wiggling your fingers; the premotor area, which is involved in planning those movements; and the prefrontal cortex, which directs executive functions like forethought, judgement, and impulse control. Short-term and working memories are first processed in the PFC as well.

Temporal lobes are located underneath your temples and behind your eyes. They are involved with encoding memories into long-term storage as well as mood stability, receptive language (reading and hearing), the reading of social cues, and mystical experiences. The temporal lobes also house the "what pathway" in the brain, which helps you recognize objects by sight and name them. You can tell "what" they are.

The parietal lobes—the top, back part of the brain—are involved with visual processing, such as seeing motion and tracking objects like a football in the air. They are involved with your sense of direction as well as your ability to know right from left, and to read and create maps in your mind. They are called the "where pathway" because they help us recognize where the things are in space. Because they are involved in spatial awareness, when the parietal lobes are damaged, people tend to have trouble catching balls, or park cars at odd angles.

The occipital lobes, located at the back of the brain, process visual information. Light enters the retinas, which sends signals to the occipital lobe on the opposite side. Light, shade, color, and basic shapes are sorted out in the occipital lobes. When these lobes are damaged, sight and perception are often affected. Visual hallucinations, illusions, or blindness sometimes occur.

Blood Flow Is Critical for a Healthy Memory

Blood is the channel that supplies cells with nutrients and clears toxins. To keep our brains sharp and healthy for as long as possible, it is critical to protect our blood vessels. In fact, brain cells don't age as quickly as once believed; research shows it is the blood vessels supporting our neurons that age.

Noting that 20 percent of the body's blood flow is used by the brain, if you have blood flow problems, you probably have them in your brain. Whatever is good for your heart is good for your brain, and whatever is bad for your heart is also bad for your brain. Not only that, but if you have blood flow problems somewhere, you probably have them everywhere. According to the Massachusetts Male Aging Study conducted from 1987 to 1989, 40 percent of forty-year-old men have erectile dysfunction. This means 40 percent of forty-year-old men also have brain dysfunction. The same study reported that 70 percent of the seventy-year-old men had erectile dysfunction, which likely means that 70 percent of the seventy-year-old men likely also have brain dysfunction. The rate rises to an alarming level in older men.

If you find yourself forgetting things and you're out of shape, getting fit could be the path back to a better memory. The reason: aerobic exercise provides greater blood flow to your brain, especially to the hippocampus, a region that's crucial to memory.

Science has revealed that reduced blood flow from the heart in old age also leads to poorer circulation in the temporal lobes, which constitute our memory "hub." In fact, if you keep your blood vessels healthy, you may be able to avoid not only memory loss and Alzheimer's disease, but also high blood pressure, heart disease, stroke, and erectile dysfunction, among other health problems. You will also have a lot more energy, and you're less likely to be overweight.

Blood Flow Risk Factors

Cardiovascular Disease

Given how important blood flow is to the brain, heart, and blood vessels, cardiovascular disease is a major risk factor for memory decline. Let us look at each potential contributor.

Plaques, the main culprit behind cardiovascular disease, is caused by a buildup of fatty deposits called plaques on the inside walls of arteries. As plaques get larger, arteries gradually narrow and can become clogged, restricting blood flow to the areas that need it. Blood flow vessels also become less elastic (also called "hardening of arteries") which raises blood pressure and makes the vessels brittle, more likely to break and cause strokes.

High levels of LDL cholesterol increase dementia risk, while high levels of HDL (good cholesterol) seem to lower it. In a four-year study of 1,037 women under eighty who had coronary artery disease, those who had elevated levels of LDL cholesterol had almost double the risk of memory loss, cognitive impairment, or dementia.

Heart attacks significantly increase the risk for future memory problems because damage to the heart decreases its ability to pump blood and keep blood flowing effectively.

Hypertension, or high blood pressure, increases the risk of memory problems. Optimal blood pressure is critical for brain health. High blood pressure and even blood pressure at the higher end of the normal range (prehypertension) are associated with lower overall brain function and blood flow to the brain. Chronically elevated pressure causes the blood vessel walls to enlarge and stiffen, making them more narrow and likely to break, much like plaques.

Strokes occur when a blood vessel breaks or a clot chokes off the blood supply to the brain, killing cells. The risk of developing dementia is six to ten times greater in a person who has had a stroke than in the general population. Even a stroke that is caused by a clot smaller than a pencil eraser increases the risk of dementia. However, risk factors such as high blood pressure, smoking, heart disease, and diabetes develop over a long time, meaning people generally have time to address these risk factors before it's too late. Recently, a Canadian researcher reported that a stroke-prevention program in Ontario had a very positive side effect: a 15.4 percent reduction in dementia over a decade in those aged eighty and over. The program included following a healthy diet, exercising, staying tobacco-free, and taking blood pressure medication, if needed.

Limited or no exercise is a major risk factor for memory loss, in large part because physical activity keeps blood vessels healthy. Exercise helps to boost a chemical called nitric oxide, which is produced in the walls of blood vessels and helps to control their shape. If blood vessel walls do not receive pulses of blood flow regularly from exercise, they begin to distort, flatten out, and limit blood flow overall. As a result, the body's tissues, including the brain, do not receive the nutrients they need or have a good mechanism to rid themselves of the toxins that build up in the body.

Strategies to Support Your Blood Flow

The strategies below can help support your overall blood flow and improve your cholesterol levels and blood pressure, all of which can cause damage to your brain.

1. **Avoid anything that hurts vascular health.** Examples include a sedentary lifestyle, caffeine, nicotine, and dehydration, all of which restrict blood flow to the brain and other organs.

2. **Seek treatment for anything that damages your blood flow.** Be serious about addressing coronary artery disease, heart arrhythmias, pre-diabetes and diabetes, prehypertension and hypertension, insomnia, sleep apnea, and drug and alcohol abuse.

3. **Lose weight if your BMI is over twenty-five.** BMI, an abbreviation for Body Mass Index, is a measure of body fat that is based on a person's height and weight. To determine your BMI, check any online BMI calculator, and learn more about this important tool.

4. **Spend ten to twenty minutes a day in deep prayer or meditation.** Both prayer and meditation have been shown to improve blood flow to the brain, particularly to the areas involved in memory and cognitive skills. Regular meditation increases blood flow to the brain, which leads to a stronger network of blood vessels in the cerebral cortex and reinforces memory capacity.

    There has been a recent surge in literature to support the effect of meditation on cognitive function and brain structures and activities. These studies have indicated that meditation alters brain activities and can have a neuroplastic effect on certain brain structures such as the prefrontal cortex, cingulate cortex, insular region, and hippocampus area.

    The impact of prayer on the brain is not as well studied as that of meditation, but some research shows that prayer influences many cortical regions, the caudate nucleus, and the dopaminergic reward system in the brain. Moreover, prayer-related activities such as religious attendance seem to have a protective effect on older adults' cognitive function.

5. **Adopt natural strategies to keep your blood pressure healthy.**

    - Eat more plant-based foods.

- Limit dairy.
- Limit salt intake.
- Eat more foods high in magnesium (e.g., pumpkin seeds) and potassium (e.g., bamboo shoots, cabbage).
- Eat more foods with blood pressure-lowering effects (e.g., broccoli, celery, garlic, chickpeas, spinach, and mushrooms).
- Eliminate alcohol, caffeine, fruit juices, and sodas (including diet sodas).
- Drink water! People who drink at least five glasses of water a day have half the risk of hypertension as those who drink fewer than two a day.
- Focus on getting seven to eight hours of sleep a night, and if you have sleep apnea, get it assessed and treated.
- Take supplements that research-based evidence has shown to lower blood pressure. These include magnesium, potassium, vitamin C and D, aged garlic, and omega-3 EPA (has inflammatory effects) and DHA (for boosting brain health).

6. ***Exercise!*** Regular exercise helps to boost nitric oxide and keep blood vessels open and flexible. Any type of exercise is great for your brain. Of course, you should check with your doctor before starting any new exercise routines.

Impact of Toxins on Your Brain and Memory

Research now shows that many people with allergies, autoimmune diseases, neurodegenerative diseases, diabetes, and cancers have one thing in common: exposure to environmental toxins. Our bodies have systems in place to get rid of toxins (through the gut, liver, kidneys, and skin), but when our detoxification systems are overwhelmed, we experience brain fog, fatigue, and life-threatening illnesses.

Toxins in any form damage the brain and increase the risk of memory problems and dementia. Common toxins associated with memory loss can be absorbed through the skin (say through a cream), ingested, or inhaled.

Check the following list to see which toxic substances you may have been exposed to, either now or in the past.

1. Toxins That Can Be Ingested or Absorbed

- BPA (bisphenol A) is found in plastics, food and drink containers, dental sealants, and the coating of cash register receipts. Nine out of ten Canadians have BPA in their bodies. Today, receipts are suspected to be a major source of our exposure to BPA and BPS, or bisphenol S, which is an organic compound.

- PCBs (polychlorinated biphenyls) are found in paints, plastics, and rubber products.

- Mercury is found in "silver" dental fillings (which are 50 percent mercury), contaminated fish, and is distributed ubiquitously in the environment.

- Lead is found in paint, pipes, aviation fuel, and lipstick.

- Cadmium is found in cigarettes, soils treated with synthetic fertilizers, and industrial waste sites. Cadmium is highly toxic and accumulates in the liver and kidneys.

- Excessive alcohol, marijuana, and various illegal drugs.

- Many pain medications, notably prescription opioids and other narcotics, or benzodiazepines for anxiety or insomnia.

- Chemotherapy can cause a long-term "brain fog" or "chemo brain."

- General anesthesia can result in long-term memory loss in some patients.

- Artificial food dyes and preservatives, including bromates, nitrates, or nitrites found in processed meats.

- Artificial sweeteners such as aspartame (blue packets), saccharin (pink), and sucralose (yellow), all are linked to toxic effects in the body.

- Pesticides include organochlorines and organophosphates. Many of them stimulate enzymes that turn calories into fat, which is where toxins are stored. In one study, people in the top 5 percent of exposure to the organochlorine pesticide DDT had a 650 percent increase in dementia.

- Apples sprayed with diphenylamine, which makes them shiny and slows discoloration but breaks down into cancer-causing nitrosamines, are associated with Parkinson's and Alzheimer's.

- Foods manufactured with plastic equipment and leaking plasticizers.

- Health and beauty products absorbed through the skin.

2. Toxins That Can Be Inhaled

- Air pollutants, whether industrial or associated with a way of life.

- Smoke from cigarettes, pipe tobacco, cigars, vaping of inhalants, second-hand smoke, all hot gases entering the lungs can be toxic.

- Automobile exhaust—carbon dioxide and monoxide, but also numerous categories of small particulate matter that come out of tailpipes.

- Gasoline fumes
- Toxins in the air near high-traffic areas
- Cleaning chemicals
- Welding, soldering fumes
- Fire retardant fumes
- Paint and solvent fumes
- Asbestos
- Aviation fumes
- Fireplace fumes
- Pesticide or herbicide residues near farms, also backyard applications
- Mold

These and other toxins may affect you without you even knowing it. In addition to those listed above, here's a closer look at everyday toxins people may encounter.

3. Toxic Beauty Products: The Price of Looking Good

The chemicals in these products are easily absorbed into your skin and transported to every organ in your body. This means that while you're trying to look good on the outside, you may be poisoning yourself on the inside.

Try to use natural products without "fragrance" and free from acrylates, aluminum, formaldehyde, oxybenzone, parabens, triclosan, polyethylene glycols, and phthalates hidden in the walls of plastic containers (go for glass wherever possible).

Products containing lead such as plastics, paint on toys, or jewelry are also of major cause for concern. Surprisingly, there are no regulations that require lead be removed from one of the most widely used cosmetics: lipstick. According to the FDA website referencing lab tests from the 1990s as well as a 2007 report from the Campaign for Safe Cosmetics, 60 percent of 33 red lipsticks of the top brands were found to contain lead.

To learn more about how to avoid buying and ingesting lead-contaminated lip products, visit *CosmeticsInfo.org* and download the Think Dirty app, which rates products on a scale of 1-10 (10=the most toxic), and scan all the products in your bathroom.

Strategies to Reduce Your Exposure to Toxins

You don't have to live like a hermit to protect your mind and save your memory. There are simple ways to avoid many toxins, and fortunately, the human body is designed to detox itself. It just needs assistance in performing the job. You can reduce your toxic load with two simple strategies: one, limit your exposure to toxins, and two, strengthen your detoxification system, especially your gut, liver, kidneys, and skin.

1. Limit Your Exposure to Toxins

- Quit smoking. Try hypnosis, nicotine patches, or bupropion (antidepressant drug to stop smoking) to kick this habit.

- Address drug and or alcohol abuse. Look for the underlying causes of why you use them. If it's due to anxiety and depression, see a doctor.

- Slowly replace "silver" dental fillings. You can opt for ceramic fillings rather than amalgams when possible.

- Reduce your consumption of toxin-contaminated foods. Buy organic (and always wash your food). One study found that concentration of selected pesticides detected in urine samples decreased by 95 percent when a family switched to organic food for two weeks.

- Always read and understand food labels. If you do not know what is in something, don't eat it or put it on your body.

- Limit or eliminate conventionally raised produce (treated with pesticides and herbicides).

- Avoid processed meat such as bacon and smoked turkey. They contain nitrosamines, which cause the liver to produce fats that are toxic to the brain.

- Limit alcohol consumption to no more than two to four servings a week; choose wine and beer over aged liquors.

- Add fiber and fiber-rich foods to your diet, which help your gastrointestinal system get rid of toxins.

- Drink eight to ten glasses of clean water a day to stay hydrated. Water helps flush toxins from your kidneys.

- Breathe clean air. Check your home for mold and eliminate it whether or not you are symptomatic.

2. Strengthen Your Detoxification Systems

- Support your gut by eating healthy foods.

- Support your skin, which is the largest organ in your body. The state of its health reflects the health of your brain.

- Work up a sweat with exercise. It's one of the best natural ways to cleanse your system. The concentration of most toxins, including arsenic, cadmium, lead, and mercury, is two to ten times higher in sweat than in blood, which makes sweating an effective detoxification process.

- Take a sauna. Saunas have been found to lower toxins in firefighters, which can be an important intervention for this at-risk group. In a follow-up study over twenty years, researchers from Finland found an inverse relationship between sauna bathing and serious memory problems.

Compared with men who had one sauna bathing session per week, those who had two to three sessions, or four to seven, were respectively 22 percent or 66 percent less likely to have dementia! In other research, those who had frequent sauna baths also had a lower incidence of sudden cardiac death and death from other causes. Saunas have also been found to help depression in cancer patients, increase feel-good endorphins and growth hormones, lower the stress hormone cortisol, and lower blood sugar.

3. The Foods That Nourish the Liver

- Green leafy vegetables contain folate, an essential detoxification nutrient.
- Protein-rich foods, such as black beans, eggs, cottage cheese, oats, turkey breasts, quinoa, guava, fish, pistachios, Greek yogurt, hemp, chia and flaxseeds, almonds, and lentils.
- Brassica, or cruciferous vegetables such as cabbage, Brussels sprouts, cauliflower, broccoli, and kale are good for detoxification.
- Oranges and tangerines
- Berries have a wide diversity of flavonoids.

4. The Foods That Nourish Your Kidneys

- Water
- Nuts and seeds such as cashews, almonds, and pumpkin seeds for magnesium
- Citrus fruits, except grapefruit
- Beet juice for circulation and endurance
- Ginger for its anti-inflammatory properties

- Garlic
- Sugar-free chocolate, which increases blood flow

5. The Foods That Nourish Your Skin

- Water
- Green tea
- Colorful fruits and vegetables for antioxidants, especially organic berries, kiwifruit, oranges, tangerines, pomegranates, broccoli, and peppers
- Avocados
- Olive oil
- Almonds, walnuts, and sunflower seeds
- Wild salmon

Remember, you should fall in love with your brain, because it runs everything in your life.

Brain health is central to all health and success in life. When your brain works right, you are happier, healthier, wealthier, and more successful in everything you do.

CHAPTER TEN

Happy Aging and Longevity Are the Greatest Wealth

Initially restricted to developed countries, population aging studies and research have become a trend in the developing world as well. However, with the rapidly advancing pace of science, one would be tempted to ask, "How close are we to stopping aging?" Can aging be reversed, or is the march of time inevitable?

As one expert in population aging at the European Molecular Biology Laboratory, Halldor Stefansson explains, "Chronic degenerative diseases—that very few people lived long enough to experience in the past—have replaced infectious and parasitic diseases as the primary cause of death." There is no doubt in my mind that scientific miracles, including age reversal technology, will be a reality soon. Our bodies will be kept biologically younger, regardless of our chronological age. The goal is to preventively target aging—the major risk factor for a wide variety of diseases and disabilities—instead of treating one disease at a time, which is very costly.

Reverse aging technology would increase not only lifespan, but health span—the period of our life for which we are healthy, happy, and productive. It would continually restore vitality and bodily function by removing the damage that is inevitably caused by the progression of life.

On the bright side, reversing the aging process is already possible for human cells and simple model organisms in scientific experiments. From yeast and worms, science has moved on to being able to extend lifespans of rats, mice, and monkeys. So, extending lifespans and reversing aging is possible in small organisms, but not yet in humans.

Genes do not play the biggest role in how you'll age. Your genes can be changed by what you eat, how much physical activity you get, and even your exposure to chemicals.

It is true that you cannot stop the process of *primary aging*. It is the law of nature that says no one and nothing can live forever. But you can slow down or reverse the process of *secondary aging*—that is, the aging process that results in worn out joints, thinning hair, and failing vision.

How to Slow Down Secondary Aging?

Life is motion, and the less we move, the more we lead an idle life. To achieve and maintain our health, we must establish a proper balance between rest and activity. If we rest too much and do not balance our rest with sufficient physical activity, fulfilling our true health potential becomes quite a task.

So, while you may not be able to turn back time, you can alter the effects of time on your body. It really is possible to slow physical and mental aging. Research has shown that people with the same chronological age may have a different "biological age." In one study published in the online journal *PNAS* (*Proceedings of the National Academy of Sciences*), 1,000 participants were examined for cognitive abilities, cardiovascular health, and other markers of fitness at the three different ages: twenty-six, thirty-two, and thirty-eight. The research plotted the slope of these individuals' biomarkers and discovered that they didn't all decline at the same rate. Some, in fact, had no slope at all, meaning they weren't aging. At thirty-eight years old, these volunteers had biological ages that ranged anywhere from younger than thirty to nearly sixty years old.

What this means for you is that factors other than genetics can influence the rate you will age. According to a study conducted at Duke University, these non-genetic factors are within your control, so read on to understand your pace of aging.

What is more shocking are the things you might be doing every day that are making you age more quickly. Hereunder is the list of those things that may be aging us faster without our knowledge.

Perfectionism

Perfectionism is a toxic side effect of our social media saturated culture, causing undue stress as we try to keep up with everyone else on the planet. Perfectionism plagues the brain with negative thoughts, which cause a release of stress hormones, which can accelerate aging. While it is fantastic to want to do your best, it is okay to have a B plus house party occasionally or take a day off to relax your head and enjoy life.

Perfectionism becomes a dominant influence because you are not free to make mistakes. This can affect your confidence as you feel that you must do everything perfectly the first time around. While it is good to be accomplishment and progress oriented, being obsessed with perfectionism is a failure and a burden on your health.

So, how to overcome perfectionism? The first step is to become aware of your perfectionist thoughts and tendencies. Take some time to pause and pay attention to your thought patterns around perfectionism. Once we are aware of how we allow perfectionism to take hold of our lives, we will be more able to alter our self-talk around this issue.

Second, focus on the positives. Wanting everything to be perfect means that we tend to fixate on the negative aspects of our work or of ourselves. However, it's important that we make a conscious effort to also recognize the good, everything you're quite satisfied with. Challenge yourself to identify three things that you do appreciate.

Third, allow yourself to make mistakes. When we give ourselves this grace, we can see that it's not the end of the world when we fail.

Mistakes are opportunities for us to learn, grow, and do better. What you might find is that mistakes are necessary to get where you want to be.

Fourth, set more reasonable goals. Perfectionists tend to set goals that are unrealistic, because of impossible standards. One way to let go of perfectionism is to set goals that are more *specific, measurable, achievable, relevant, attainable,* and *time-bound* or SMART. We will feel much less stressed and more confident in our ability to reach our goals when they are realistic and challenging in a healthy way.

Fifth, learn how to receive criticism. People who are perfectionists tend to have low self-esteem because they take criticism personally. Try to recognize that healthy criticism can be helpful and is normal because it can allow us to be better.

Sixth, lower the pressure you put on yourself. Remember that the person who pressures you the most is yourself. Be kind to yourself and practice self-acceptance by lowering unrealistic standards you set for yourself. If you are still motivated and doing your best, you're doing just fine. There is no such thing as "perfect," but we can be proud of doing our best.

Lastly, therapy can help with our anxiety around perfectionism. Cognitive behavioral therapy (CBT) can help people struggling with perfectionism to reframe their thoughts. Therapy can also help you to better understand the deeper reason behind feeling the pressure to be perfect. If you find that you're still struggling, therapy may be a good option to give you even more tools to overcome perfectionism.

Cynical Hostility

A cynic is someone who doesn't trust other people. He or she may believe that behind every good deed there is usually a selfish or an impure motive. So, when a friendly neighbor greets a cynic in the morning, he or she starts doubting the neighbor's intentions. And hostility is bitterness and unfriendliness. But if you want to stop aging fast, you better start trusting people and being good to them.

So, how to stop being cynical? Remove judgement from your

life. Allow people to find their own way and respect that they are on their own journey. Judgement blinds us to the truth sometimes and judging less will keep us from finding fault in others.

Second, practice loving and kindness. This is a simple practice where you can express your intentions for the day. Ask for a day of peace, love, hope, kindness, friendliness and pleasant experiences with the same. This will begin to help you think more positively.

Third, consider the people you surround yourself with. After all, it's hard to break habits when everyone around you is doing the same thing. So, if you find that many of your friends or family members are cynical too, either try to get them on board to change as well or start surrounding yourself with people who have a more positive attitude.

Fourth, connect with more well-meaning people. One who has determined to be free from cynicism will have to allow themselves to feel the discomfort of being cynical again. After a while, that discomfort will turn into curiosity, excitement, and reinforcement that there is no need to be cynical.

Rumination

The process of continuously thinking about the same thoughts, which tend to be sad or dark, is called rumination. Most people live in the present, but some of us are still stuck in the past. Ruminating or thinking regretfully about the past may be bad for your health. If you are beating yourself up over an unfortunate incident in the past, it could cause more depression and shortening of the telomere or shortening of your lifespan. So, if your constant thinking cannot do you any good, stop! Don't get sucked into a rumination state.

But how to address ruminating thoughts? When you realize you're starting to ruminate, finding a distraction can break your thought cycle. Look around you, quickly choose something else to do, and don't give it a second thought. Consider:

- Calling a friend or family member
- Watching a movie

- Reading a book

- Walking around your neighborhood

- Second, instead of going over the same negative thought repeatedly, take that thought and plan to address it. In your head, outline each step you need to take to address the problem, or write it down on a piece of paper. Be realist and as specific as possible with your expectations. Doing this will disrupt your rumination and will help you move forward in the attempt to get a negative thought out of your head once and for all.

- Third, work on enhancing your self-esteem. Many people who ruminate report difficulties with self-esteem. In fact, a lack of self-esteem can be associated with increased rumination. Some people may choose to work on the enhancement of their self-esteem in psychotherapy. As you enhance your self-esteem, self-efficacy may also be enhanced, and you may find that you're better able to control rumination.

- Fourth, talk to a friend. Ruminating thoughts can make you feel isolated. Talk about your thoughts with a friend who can give you perspective rather than ruminate with you.

Wandering Thoughts

Mind wandering is the experience of thoughts not remaining on a single topic for a long period of time, particularly when people are engaged in an attention-demanding task. Scientific evidence says that mind wandering can be a sign of unhappiness.

Taking baby steps may come in handy. Practice meditation, be grateful, take good care of your body, and challenge your negative thoughts as they crop up in your mind. Always remember what the British novelist Roald Dahl said: "A person who has good thoughts cannot ever be ugly. You can have a wonky nose and a crooked mouth

Chapter Ten: Happy Aging and Longevity Are the Greatest Wealth

and a double chin and stick-out teeth, but if you have good thoughts, it will shine out of your face like sunbeams, and you'll always look lovely."

Giving your mind more to do reduces distractions. Research by Nilli Lavie at University College London has found that adding deliberate distractions such as a bit of background noise reduces distractibility. Her "load theory" proposes this is because attention is a limited resource, so if you fill all the attentional "slots" in your mind, it leaves no room for other distractions.

Stress

In a landmark study published in online journal *PNAS*, stress was shown to shorten lifespan. People with the highest stress levels had shorter telomeres, or shorter lifespans. It was if these people were a decade older than those in the lowest stress category, the study's authors say.

It's natural to have daily demands and deadlines, but if you are constantly running from one thing to the next, caught in a whirlwind of busyness, you are aging yourself faster. Stress hormones cause your blood vessels to constrict, and chronic stress increases your risk of heart disease, high blood pressure, cancer, and stroke. It can also cause or exacerbate mental health problems.

Learning to manage your stress takes practice, but you can. There are few ways to make it easier, and their first way is to exercise. Working out regularly is one of the best ways to relax your body and mind. Plus, exercise will improve your mood. But you must do it often for it to pay off. So how much should you exercise every week? Work up to two hours and thirty minutes of moderately intense exercise, like brisk walks, or seventy-five minutes of a more vigorous exercise, like swimming laps, jogging, or other sports.

The second way is to relax your muscles. When you are stressed, your muscles get tense. You can help loosen them up on your own and refresh your body by:

- Stretching

- Enjoying a massage

- Taking a hot bath or shower
- Getting a good night's sleep

The third way is to slow down. Modern life is so busy, and sometimes we just need to slow down and chill out. Look at your life and find small ways you can do that. For example:

- When you are driving on the highway, switch to the slow lane so you can avoid road rage.
- Break down big jobs into smaller ones. For example, don't try to answer all one hundred emails if you don't have to—just answer a few of them.

The fourth way is to set time for hobbies. It doesn't need to be a ton of time—even fifteen to twenty minutes will do. Relaxing hobbies include things like:

- Reading
- Watching movies
- Doing puzzles
- Playing cards and board games

Habits That May Make You Live Longer

Don't fall for the myth that growing older automatically means you are not going to feel good anymore. It is true that aging involves physical changes, but it doesn't have to mean discomfort and disability. While not all illness or pain is unavoidable, many of the physical challenges associated with aging can be overcome or drastically mitigated by exercising, eating right, and taking care of yourself.

As already mentioned in the previous pages of this book, physical activity is crucial to our well-being because it helps offset many of the effects of aging. According to MedlinePlus, exercising regularly can

Chapter Ten : Happy Aging and Longevity Are the Greatest Wealth

improve your balance, help keep you mobile, improve your mood by reducing feelings of anxiety and depression, and contribute to better cognitive functioning. This means, the best way to slow aging is to stay in great shape. Physical activity has many benefits and is essential for living a healthy life into old age and being physically active on a daily basis improves your quality of life.

The following are simple ways you can exercise without a trainer:

Dancing

Whether you fancy the rumba, cha-cha-cha, polka, twist, or ballet, bop, shimmy, Jazzercise, square-dancing, or folk dancing, the idea is to go, flow, rock, sway, turn-strut, swing, and sweep to your favorite tunes. Without even noticing it, you'll give your body and bones an exhilarating workout.

Walking

Walking is perfect because it's an activity that is beneficial to the bones but doesn't feel like work. You should walk for at least thirty minutes, five times a week, for the exercise to be effective. Walk with your spouse or a friend. It's a wonderful way to socialize and share your thoughts.

Walking is an easy and accessible form of exercise, whatever age you are. Walking can help you build stamina, burn excess calories, and make your heart healthier. You can fit walking around your schedule or head out for a stroll on a whim. It's free to do and has many health benefits. Even a fifteen-minute wander to the shops can benefit your physical and mental well-being.

Many studies link moderate daily exercise, such as walking, to an improved mental outlook and reduced risk of depression and anxiety. People who walk to work say they arrive at the office feeling energized and alert, without an artificial boost from caffeine.

Bicycling

Bicycling for exercising or commuting is a guaranteed way to engage in moderate physical activity. Bicycling burns about five hundred calories per hour. It exercises your heart, lungs, and muscles. It tones and firms your arms, legs, shoulders, and buttocks. It burns fat and increases metabolism. It helps you lose weight without dieting. It builds your immune system and makes you less likely to get sick. It reduces the risk of heart attack and stroke.

Bicycling is also considered low-impact exercise, so you won't damage your knees or other joints. It may even help you live longer. There are more simple things such as washing your face before you go to bed or applying sunscreen every day, that may contribute to slowing your aging process.

Wash Your Face before Bed

You know you're supposed to do it, but sometimes you just don't. Experts stress that failure to wash your face at the end of the day is a major missed opportunity for the skin to regenerate while you sleep. Skin renews itself overnight, so if you want to change the way your skin functions, and looks, take a few minutes at night to wash your face.

Apply Sunscreen Every Day

It doesn't matter if you're not hitting the beach or spending all day outside, you'll still need to apply sunscreen every day. The sun is the biggest factor in aging skin, so if you don't want wrinkles before your time, make sure you're applying a lotion with an SPF of at least thirty every morning. You should put it on before any makeup or other products.

Exercising Outdoors Is Good for You

Studies show that exercising outdoors or in nature is even better for your mental health. Getting some fresh air when out for a walk or bike ride leaves you feeling energized, positive, and ready to take on whatever life throws at you. And it helps to calm you if you're feeling tense or angry.

A Healthy Mouth Is Healthy Aging

There is a connection between a healthy mouth and healthy aging. Research has shown poor dental health is linked to age-related problems such as cardiovascular disease, stroke, and diabetes, possibly because bacteria from oral infections may get into the blood and increase inflammation in other parts of the body. In addition, recent studies indicate that gum disease may be linked to a higher risk of dementia and Alzheimer's. Although these connections are still under study, it's worth keeping your teeth healthy and possibly preventing these age-related diseases with good dental habits.

Your teeth are one of the first places to show the wear and tear of aging. You should protect your youthful smile by not only flossing and brushing, but also by seeing your dentist for regular checkups. Investing in whitening strips or other cosmetic procedures can take years off your looks.

Keep Your Gut Healthy

Research has found the collection of "good" bacteria in your intestines, called the *gut microbiome,* may have implications on how your body ages; it may even protect you from some age-related diseases such as dementia. In one study published in the journal *Cell,* the presence of certain gut bacteria slowed the rate of aging in worms, which may lead to anti-aging bacteria treatments for humans in the future.

According to Dr. Steven Gundry, and author of *The Longevity Paradox: How to Die Young at a Ripe Old Age,* about 70 percent of your immune system resides in your gut, so maintaining gut health as you age is important to your overall health. Among other things, your gut provides protection from infections, regulates your metabolism, supports your immune system, and promotes a healthy gastrointestinal function. To encourage healthy gut flora as you age, you should choose prebiotic and probiotic foods such as fiber-rich fruits, vegetables, kefir, yogurt, sauerkraut, and kimchi. Exercise, fiber, and fluids can also help keep things moving through your digestive tract.

Healthy Digestion

Because older people, especially those who are overweight, are prone to acid reflux, you may think of your stomach acid as the enemy. But you need a healthy supply of digestive acids to absorb B12 to keep your brain sharp. According to gastroenterologist Dr. Mark Epstein, acid-reducing medicines, like metformin for diabetes, can decrease the absorption of nutrients such as vitamin B12.

To prevent this, supplements and fortified foods may be necessary. You can also get B12 from fish, eggs, poultry, and dairy products.

Avoid Salt

Excess salt bleeds calcium out of the body via urine, and a single teaspoon of salt a day can cause bone mass to decrease by 1.5 percent a year. Osteoporosis may join the growing list of reasons people should reduce salt. Good news, a salt substitute, called Salt Free, is available in Canada and several more countries.

Avoid Alcoholism

While men, under normal conditions, don't suffer the damage of osteoporosis until their eighties (which is beyond their current estimated life expectancy), there's evidence that alcoholism could put them in the same boat as women. A study of ninety-six chronic alcoholic men at the Veterans Administration Hospital, in Hines, Illinois, determined that 47 percent had evidence of bone loss, and what was even more telling, 31 percent were under forty years old.

Drink Red Wine in Moderation

Studies reveal that resveratrol, the antioxidant present in the grape skin, has both anti-aging and heart-healthy benefits. Flavonoids like anthocyanins that give the wine its rich red colour provides many benefits to your body. When it comes to aging and alcohol, there is a fine line between protective and problematic. Some studies have found that the occasional glass of wine may offer some anti-aging benefits, but more than two a day is associated with a decrease in lifespan.

Red wine is good for overall health, including protection from heart disease, and decreasing inflammation. It also improves blood lipid levels and reduces the risk of dementia.

Drink Coffee in Moderation

To the relief of caffeine lovers everywhere, here is how to live longer without sacrificing your favorite drink. Your daily cup of coffee may have health benefits that could extend your life. Some research indicates moderate coffee intake may fight against type 2 diabetes and may even reduce the risk of dementia and heart disease. A moderate amount of coffee is generally defined as three to five cups a day, or an average 400 mg of caffeine, according to the Dietary Guidelines for Americans.

A study from Harvard found that those who regularly drank coffee lived longer than those who didn't.

Eat Carrots

These vegetables supply a hearty helping of beta carotene, which is a precursor to vitamin A, a critical nutrient for skin health that also slows aging. As an antioxidant, it helps fend off aging for your entire body too. And as an additional bonus, beta carotene warms your complexion, and a beta carotene rich glow has been scientifically proven to be more attractive than a suntan.

Vitamin C Foods

In a study published in the *American Journal of Clinical Nutrition*, researchers found that people who ate vitamin C rich foods had fewer wrinkles and less age-related dry skin than those who did not.

Dark Chocolate

One delicious treat that may even have anti-aging properties is dark chocolate. Research has suggested it may protect against fatal heart attacks, and one study found that participants who drank hot chocolate every day for twenty weeks even had a younger-looking skin texture, possibly due to its anti-inflammatory effects. Who doesn't love chocolate? It satisfies cravings, it is low in sugar, offers fiber, and contains antioxidants.

Use Glutathione—the Master Antioxidant

Many scientists refer to glutathione as the mother of all antioxidants or, sometimes, the master of all antioxidants. And the glutathione does quite a bit of what we might call "mothering." It makes sure that the little ones—like vitamins C, beta carotene, and other antioxidants—are taken care of after they have donated their electrons to neutralize unstable atoms or free radicals that cause illness and aging. When glutathione replaces those donations with its own electrons, it's like the selfless mom who, when the temperature drops, gives up her sweater to the ten-year-old who left hers at home.

In a different sense, glutathione acts in a mastery fashion. As the only antioxidant that can recycle itself as well as the antioxidant that decides when to sacrifice its brethren by snatching their electrons. It runs the show. And that is essential, because no other antioxidant can go all the places in the body that glutathione can go. As you might know, we age prematurely because of damage done by free radicals to our body.

Glutathione in a nutshell is an antioxidant, a detoxifier, and the second most abundant molecule in the body. It's your first line of defense in fighting free radicals, makes it possible for your body to eliminate toxins, and supports overall cellular health. Oh, and by doing this, it also helps defend against disease and *slow down aging*.

The good news is that the body can both absorb already-made glutathione from food and make glutathione from its building blocks. I recommend you eat plenty of the following foods with the highest concentration of glutathione.

Fruit

- Avocado (about ¾ fruit) 20.6 mg

- Strawberries (about ¾ cup, halved) 6.9 mg
- Grapefruit (about 6 sections) 6.5 mg
- Cantaloupe (about 1 large wedge) 6.1 mg
- Papaya (about 1 cup, 1-inch pieces) 5.8 mg
- Watermelon (about ¾ cup, sliced) 5 mg
- Peaches (about ¾ cup, sliced) 5 mg
- Oranges (about 6 sections) 4.8 mg

Vegetables

- Asparagus (about 5 large spears) 21.8 mg
- Spinach (raw) (about 3 cups) 11.4 mg
- Okra (8-9 pods) 11.3 mg
- Winter squash (about 1 scant cup, cubed) 11 mg
- Potatoes (with skin) (about ½ medium) 11 mg
- Tomatoes (about 3 large, thick slices) 7.5 mg
- Carrots (about 2 small) 5.9 mg
- Spinach (cooked) (about 2 cups) 5.7 mg

Meat, Poultry, Fish

- Pork chop (about 3 ½ ounces) 18.9 mg
- Steak (about 3 ½ ounces) 12.3 mg
- Hamburger (about 3 ½ ounces) 11.8 mg
- Chicken (about 3 ½ ounces) 7.7 mg
- Fish (cod) (about 4 ounces) 5.7 mg

Stop Eating before You Are Full

Japanese people in general, and the people living in Okinawa in particular, are the longest living in the world. Why? They eat lots of vegetables and fish and stop eating before they are full—this tradition is called *"hara hachi bu"* in Japan. Eating this way works for the Japanese, so it can work for you too. Also try bitter lemon, an important part of healthy food in Okinawa for centuries. This is notable because the older people in Okinawa appear to be the healthiest elderly population in the world.

Enjoy Sunshine and Connect with Nature

Anyone wondering how to live longer needs to hear the benefits of vitamin D, "the sunshine vitamin," that helps keep your bones strong, and it may also help protect against age-related conditions like heart disease and cancer.

Getting thirty minutes of sun a day should be adequate for vitamin D production. Of course, that is not necessarily through sunbathing but by being outside wearing normal clothing. You can also get vitamin D in foods such as fatty fish, egg yolks, and fortified foods, including cereals.

There are countless benefits to spending time outdoors, but when it comes to aging, stress relief caused by being in nature can be incredibly beneficial. Green and blue spaces promote feelings of renewal, restoration, and inner peace.

Travel the World if You Can

Nothing makes you feel like you want to stick around planet Earth a little longer than traveling in some of life's most inspiring sights, tastes, and sounds.

Perhaps one of the most important ways to create meaning in your life as you age is to visit different regions of the world if you can, because we don't often get to explore the world when we are young. So, when we get older, we have a chance to do that and experience moments that truly touch our soul. Science says that simply checking out on a vacation could be one way to live longer.

One large study of middle-aged men at high risk for heart disease found those who took annual vacations lived longer than those who did not. Another study had similar results in women.

Physical Intimacy and Sex

You can have a healthy and rewarding sex life at any age. Sex can be a powerful emotional experience and a great exercise in improving health, and it's certainly not for the young only. The need for intimacy is ageless. And studies now confirm that no matter what your gender, you can enjoy sex for as long as you wish.

Although there are some obstacles to sex as we age (vaginal dryness in women; erectile dysfunction in men), continuing to get busy could help expand our lives. People who remain sexually active as they age do tend to live longer. Naturally, sex at seventy or eighty may not be like it is at twenty or thirty, but it can be enjoyable.

As an older adult, you may feel wiser than you were in your earlier years and know what works best for you when it comes to your sex life. Older people often have a great deal more self-confidence and self-awareness and feel released from the unrealistic ideals of youth and the prejudices of others. And with children grown and work less demanding, couples are better able to relax and enjoy one another without the old distractions.

Old age doesn't necessarily kill your libido. Impotence and reduced libido are related to normally preventable medical conditions like high blood pressure, heart disease, diabetes, and depression. The solution is keeping yourself in shape. Something as simple as lifting weights a couple of times a week can improve your sex life.

Shirley Zussman, EdD, who believes that sex should be no less important than your exercise routine, suggests you schedule time with your sweetheart, even if it means reordering your priorities, like foregoing your French lessons or hiring someone to help clean the house. You may just find that a little romance in the morning will put pep in your step, a smile on your face, and give you extra energy all day.

At the end of your morning sex, make it routine to hug your soulmate. Receiving a hug first thing in the morning would light up his or her entire day. Hugging relaxes muscles, releases tension in the body, and soothes aches by increasing circulation in the soft tissues.

Nurture Relationships

If you're in a relationship, treat your partner like they're the most fantastic person on the planet. Even though you're no longer in the "young love" phase of your relationship, that's no reason for romance to wane. In fact, according to a recent national poll on health aging conducted by the University of Michigan, 76 percent of the participants, who ranged from sixty-five to eighty years old, believed sex was important at any age. So instead of buying into the myth that intimacy declines with age, consider all the positives that could help your relationship flourish in your golden years: more privacy, more time, less stress, and more opportunities for romantic getaways. And if you are not currently dating but want to be, there's no reason to let age stop you from doing it.

Anti-Aging Benefits of Friendship

Friends are not only good for remembering your birthday, or picking you up from the airport, friendships also have powerful anti-aging benefits. Studies have shown that people with a strong social network and satisfying relationships tend to lead longer, happier lives. Whenever possible or occasionally, consider spending a night out with friends instead of an evening on the couch with Netflix.

Having strong relationships predicts a 50 percent increased chance of longevity. Research suggests that connecting with others in a meaningful way helps us enjoy better mental and physical health, even speeding up recovery from disease.

Be Generous and Supportive to Others

Connecting with others is a great stress reliever, which can help your long-term health. And the best way to harness these benefits is by focusing not only on yourself, but also on others. A study conducted with an elderly population showed that those who engaged in helping and supporting others ended up living longer lives.

The health benefits of helping others don't just apply to people you know. Research has also found that volunteering is not only good for you, but a study from the University of Michigan showed that volunteerism predicts a longer life.

Stay Young at Heart

You are only as old as you feel and feeling young may help you live longer. Research found that people who felt three years younger had a lower death rate than those who felt their age or older. Other explanations could be that our attitude towards age affects how healthy we live.

Age Gratefully

We've heard about aging gracefully, but it's important to age gratefully as well, which means, if you think of a long life in positive terms, you are more likely to have one! Research has proven that cultivating gratitude increases well-being. Conscious aging is sometimes referred to as vital aging, successful aging, or grateful aging, and the science behind it says that we can live longer by learning to become appreciative of the aging process.

Maintain a Positive Attitude

Having a positive attitude about aging, maintaining a purpose, and staying socially engaged may help slow the physical and mental aging process. One study revealed that the people with a positive attitude lived 7.5 years longer than pessimists, regardless of health.

A study from Harvard looked at how levels of optimism affected different health problems and found the most optimistic people had a 16 percent lower risk of death from cancer, a 38 percent lower risk of death from heart and respiratory disease, and 39 percent lower risk of dying from stroke. The researchers believe that having a positive outlook makes you more likely to engage in healthy behaviors like exercising and eating right, but that it might also be connected to lower levels of inflammation.

Maintaining a positive attitude and remaining connected socially not only helps us prevent depression, but also to better cope with health conditions, and even live longer.

Finding a Meaning, Purpose, and Joy

A key ingredient in the recipe for longevity is the continuing ability to find meaning and joy in life. As you age, your life will change, and you'll gradually lose things that previously occupied your time and gave your life purpose. For example, your job may change, you may eventually retire from your career, your children may leave home, or other friends and family may move far away. But this is not the time to stop moving forward. Later life can be an exciting new adventure if you let it.

When you have something to live for, you just might end up sticking around a little longer. And science backs this up. London University College conducted a study of 9,000 people aged over sixty-five and found that those who had the greatest sense of purpose in their life were 30 percent less likely to die during the next eight years than those with the lowest sense of purpose. Studies show that creating meaning in life brings happiness and greater health.

Doing what you like to do is good for your overall health and contributes to stress reduction. Having goals for the future can promote your physical well-being.

Control What You Can

If someone is dreading aging, the most important thing they can do is take the best care of their health. Once you know you are doing all you can to live a long and productive life, obsessing over the opposite is counterproductive, unfortunate, and premature death.

Shift your mindset to acknowledge that while some things might be out of your control (like genetics), other things are. Get regular checkups. Speak with a doctor if you find yourself very stressed or struggling with a mental health concern. Make time for self-care activities, like joyful movement and eating in a way that makes you feel your best.

Use Your Life Experiences

Aging is about using your experiences, tools for healthful living, and wisdom to make the journey into your golden years the most fulfilling of your life.

Live in the Now

With age and wisdom come a whole lot of memories. You should do your best to avoid serious thoughts on the ups and downs over the course of life, such as relationship struggles, health challenges, or financial hardships. One of the best things you can do as you age is to stay as present as possible. This will not only help you fully live your life, but also give you some substantial mental health benefits.

Living in the past can be dangerous and will hold you back. Do what you must and deal with it or accept it. Don't flush it away, and don't deny it, but find a way to move on. While it might not be possible to wipe your memory clean of past hardships or painful experiences, mindfulness can help you detach your past from your present.

Stay Inspired

In tandem with finding your purpose, it's important to stay inspired each day. If you read a book about the treasury of wit and wisdom, or inspirational quotes every day for ten minutes, it adds up and can change your whole outlook on life.

I suggest having role models who emulate aging gracefully, particularly for anyone struggling to see aging in a positive way. For example, Fauja Singh became the world's oldest marathon runner at the age of one hundred after completing his very first marathon at the age of eighty-nine.

Stay Connected

Although we hear a lot about the negative aspects of social media, it not only keeps us connected, but it is also essential for long-term well-being. Researchers at Claremont Graduate University say interacting on social media increases oxytocin, the "feel good hormone." Keeping connected online with social media can enhance longevity if your time is spent with supportive and meaningful activities.

One of the greatest challenges of aging is maintaining your support network. Staying connected isn't always easy as you grow older—even for those who have always had an active social life. Staying social can have the most impact on your health as you age. Having an array of people you can turn to for company and support as you age is a buffer against loneliness, depression, disability, hardship, and loss.

On the bright side, scientists are teaching us why we age, and what we can do to slow down and even reverse the aging process. Through their efforts, we now know that aging begins at the cellular level with free radical damage, and that antioxidant vitamins, minerals, enzymes, and exercise can prevent such destruction.

As this information reaches the public, more and more people are attempting to turn back the clock by eating better, supplementing their diets, reducing stress, and increasing their physical activity. In fact, with today's knowledge, and increasingly positive attitudes, extending our healthful years to equal those of the Hunza tribe of the Himalayan highlands and the Okinawans in Japan is possible.

Today more than ever before, the ability to die young at a ripe old age is indeed a possibility that is available to us all.

Conclusion

Everyone is searching for happiness and meaning in their lives. You are not alone in your journey. Remember—your greatest happiness is already inside you. You can achieve whatever you want, whenever you want, when you let your happiness out. Your ability to create, achieve,

Chapter Ten : Happy Aging and Longevity Are the Greatest Wealth

strive, love, risk, and dare is what drives your happiness. They say you get wiser as you get older. Assuming that you are already older, get wise now. Start applying the concepts you've learned in this book to make changes today. When you do, you'll start leading a successful life.

You can achieve success with the abilities and tools you already have. However, tools are powerless without action. This is your time to shine, and only you control your spotlight. Find your path, embrace excellence, and go all in. Keep moving. No one is going to do this for you.

Life mastery requires an understanding of multiple concepts that connect to and provide mental models for dealing with life's situations. Continual success—the ability to design the life and lifestyle you truly want to live—is the consequence of a series of good decisions. At the same time, continual failure to achieve your desired life and lifestyle is the consequence of a series of bad decisions. How do we improve the quality of our decisions? By understanding the concepts that contribute to a successful life and applying mental models that relate to those concepts.

The universe is benevolent. It wants you to succeed, but it gives you tests to pass so you don't fail at the next level. When you shift your perception about failure, you will realize, like me, that it is truly possible to succeed in old age.

Don't just be inspired by *why*. Be inspired by *how*. How you do something will guarantee your success. If you bring passion, joy, and enthusiasm to whatever you want to get results in, your success will also be guaranteed.

Find something you care about and commit deeply to it. To succeed, you will have to go all the way. And when you attempt to go all the way, you will sometimes fail, but these are lessons. This is important. Failures are temporary, and failure is the only way to succeed. Make mistakes, but don't make the same mistake more than twice.

And remember this: You cannot succeed if you quit. Quitting comes down to perspective in most cases. Often, a setback is simply a reminder to change course, to take a detour. Not to stop, but to change strategy, change plans, change perspective. At this point, it's about time you think differently. Don't accept the status quo. Change things. Push forward. You don't have to be a genius. You just must believe that you can change your world. You can change your life. Not to be rich, but to live rich. Look within and make the decision to replace negative thinking with positive thoughts. Accept your flaws, your past, and your current situation. Know that you won't be perfect with every step and every decision. You will make mistakes, but you will not disappoint yourself if you make the choice to commit, trust yourself, and enjoy the journey.

Success is a mindset. Your mentality becomes your reality. Success begets more success, and it can snowball quickly. What you appreciate, appreciates. In the investment world this is called "compound returns."

Just remember not to over-celebrate your success and overspend like lottery winners who tend to return to their original level of happiness once the novelty has worn off. The point is you are in control of your own happiness and no amount of money is going to solve that. Because, as the saying goes, wherever you go, there you are. Control what you can control, enjoy everything else along the way.

Dear reader, I fear you may have hesitated to buy this book, thinking it was written by a young man trying to make quick money off the elderly. This is not the case. I wanted to do my part in making the world a better place, leave a legacy, and share my rich experience dating back to a few years after the end of World War II.

I hope I inspired a new way of thinking, and helped you tap into your creative brain. I truly believe you now know that good health is the first wealth, and that Humor, gratitude, and happiness are part and parcel of a long life.

As I depart, I want to express my gratitude to you. When I decided to write a book for older adults and seniors and self-publish it, I didn't know if anyone would care to read it, but here you are. I'd love to stay in touch and hear your stories and feedback. If you want to reach out to me directly, don't hesitate to email me at amonsuccessforseniors@gmail.com. If you enjoyed *How to Succeed After 55*, it would mean the

Chapter Ten : Happy Aging and Longevity Are the Greatest Wealth

world to me if you left an honest review on Amazon or Good reads to help other people discover it.

I wish you nothing but success, good health, happiness and long life.

Acknowledgments

I would like to thank those who taught me how to write, from my father to all the others who encouraged me to express. I am particularly indebted to Paula LaRocque and Joanna Penn, whose books were a valuable source of guidance and inspiration in making this contribution to the world.

To Matt Swann Creative, thank you for your eye-catching cover design. And to the entire Aaxel Author Services team, thank you for your beautiful interior design. In addition, I gratefully acknowledge my talented indexer, Judith Nylvek. Thank you for putting much care into writing a quality and valuable index.

Finally, I wish to express my heartfelt gratitude to my amazing editor, Alexa Nazzaro. At each stage of the editorial process, you have been insightful, meticulous, and unflagging in your enthusiasm that brought this book to completion.

Thank you all and God bless all of you.

Index

AARP, 103
accounting, 41–42
achievements
    compounding development effect and, 23–25
    emotional contagion and, 19–21
    personal, 17
    responsibility for, 18–19
    standards of excellence for, 25–27
achievers, high, 18
action, taking, 47–50
action plan, 26–27
activities, 176–178, 184–186
advice, negative, 22–23

aging
- activity and, 176–178, 184–186
- attitudes to, 184–190
- gratitude and, 187
- health and, 179–184
- process of, 169–170
- relationships and, 185–187
- slowing, 170–176
- success and, 190–193

air pollutants, 163
alcoholism, 180
Allen, Tom, 14
Allrecipes.com, 80
anesthesia, 163
Angelou, Maya, 151
antioxidants, 180–183
Art of Living, The (Peale), 60
artificial sweeteners, 163
asking questions, 59
athleticism, 133–134
attention, lack of, 174–175
author, about, 5–7

Bach, David, *Start Late, Finish Rich*, 70
"Basic Online Skills," 101
beauty products, 164–165
Becoming Warren Buffett (HBO documentary), 86
beliefs, 26, 43–44

Index

bicycling, 177
Biden, Joe, 14
bisphinol A (BPA), 162
blood flow, 157–161
BMI (body mass index), 160
body clock, 56
body mass index (BMI), 160
Bonaparte, Napoleon, 61
BPA (bisphinol A), 162
brain health
    blood flow and, 157–161
    detoxification and, 165–168
    food for, 153
    functions of regions and, 156–157
    memory problems and, 153–154
    memory rescue and, 154–156
    toxins and, 161–165
Branson, Richard, 151
British Royal Academy of Arts, 110
budgeting, 64–65, 75–76, 79
Buffett, Suzie, 83, 86
Buffett, Warren, 42, 82–87, 95
Buffett: The Making of an American Capitalist (Lowenstein), 86

cadmium, 162
cardiovascular disease, 158–159
career advancement, humor and, 110–113
Carnegie, Dale, *How To Win Friends and Influence People*, 114

CARP (Canadian Association for Retired Persons), 103
carrots, 181
cash, paying with, 69–70
change, starting, 10–12
chemotherapy, 162
Chen, Lung Hung, 133
chocolate, dark, 181
cholesterol, 158–159
classes. see continuing education
coffee, 181
comedy, styles and techniques of, 117–120
comparison shopping, 74
complacency, 62
compounding development effect, 23–25
compounding interest, 24
Connecticut Distance Learning Consortium, 101
consumer debt, 66–67
consumption, culture of, 88
contagion, emotional, 19–21
continuing education, 68
Cook, Tim, 85
cosmetic dentistry, 115
Craigslist, 73
critical thinking, 40
cynicism, 172–173

Dahl, Roald, 174
dancing, 177

debt, 70–71
decision making, 38, 40
detoxification, 165–168
dietary guidelines, 160–161, 180–184
    see also foods; meal planning
digestion, 180
digital age, 98–102
discontentment, 44–45
Dweck, Carol, 30, 109

Easterlin paradox, 149
eBay, 73
Edison, Thomas, 15, 31
education, continuing, 68
education vs. learning, 95
Einstein, Albert, 15
emotional contagion, 19–21
empathy, 46, 134
employment, finding, 68–69
empowerment, 27–30
endorphins, 146
energy, 55, 133
entrepreneurship, 105
evaluation, of self, 26–27
Evernote, 103
excellence, 25–27
exercising, 147, 159, 161, 176–178
exhaust, 163

expectations, standards of, 25
expenses, unnecessary, 70–71
experiences, as resources, 11
experiential learning, 94–95

Facebook, 101
failures, 31, 36
fees, 78–79
fexibility, 38–39
finances
    compounding development effect and, 24
    management of, 63–67, 79–87, 89–91
    personal, 11
    see also budgeting; debt; investing; money
financial security, 63–64
    see also wealth
fitness, 11
fixed mindset, 31–32
food dyes, 163
foods
    for brain health, 153
    with glutathione, 182–183
    healthy, 165–168
    see also dietary guidelines; meal planning
Forbes, B.C., 51
Franklin, Benjamin, 53, 95
friendships, 186
frontal lobes, 156

fumes, 164

G. Raymond Chang School of Continuing Education, 94
Gandhi, Mahatma, 142
Gates, Bill, 84
GCFLearnFree.org, 101
glutathione, 182–183
goals
    aging and, 89
    desired, 26
    strategies to achieve, 42–47
    talking about, 49–50
Google, 80
gratitude
    aging and, 187
    brain and, 134
    happiness and, 130–131
    importance of, 131–136
    practicing, 127–130
    purpose of, 126–127
    success and, 136
growth mindset, 30–32, 109
Gundry, Steven, *Longevity Paradox: How to Die Young at a Ripe Old Age*, 179

halo effect, 115
"ham drawing contest," 110
happiness

causes of, 143–145
　　　definitions of, 141–143
　　　global pursuit of, 149
　　　gratitude and, 130–132
　　　humor and, 107–109
　　　joyful living and, 60–62
　　　measures of, 150–151
　　　positivity and, 145–148
　　　science of, 139–140
　　　searching for, 190–193
　　　spending money and, 87–88
　　　success and, 37, 140–141
hardships, 134–135
Harvard Business Review, 111
health
　　　aging and, 170–171, 173, 175, 177, 179–189
　　　fitness and, 11
　　　mental state and, 133
　　　psychological, 136
　　　see also brain health
health care needs, 89
heart attacks, 158
help, asking for, 50–52
Hess, Edward, *Learn or Die*, 104
high blood pressure, 158–159
Hill, Napoleon, 61
　　　Law of Success, The, 53
　　　Think and Grow Rich, 53

Index

housing, 90–91
How of Happiness, The (Lyubomirsky), 142
How To Win Friends and Influence People (Carnegie), 114
how-to books, 101
Hsieh, Tony, 151
humor
    developing a sense of, 116–124
    happiness and, 107–109
    success and, 109–116
Humor Advantage, The (Kerr), 108
hypertension, 158–159

Idealist.org, 102
information age, 100–102
interest, 24, 71–72
intestinal health, 179–184
intimacy, 185–186
introduction, 1–3
investing, 76–77

Jackson, Phil, 57
jokes, 117–118, 121–123
Jordan, Michael, 57

Kerr, Michael, 113
    Humor Advantage, The, 108
Kijiji.ca, 73
kindness, 146

Kingdom of Bhutan, 149
knowledge, 96–98

Lamb, Charles, 61
Latte Factor, 70
laughing, 121–124
Law of Success, The (Hill), 53
lead, 162, 164–166
Learn or Die (Hess), 104
    learning
    benefits of, 104–105
    lifelong, 94–96
    resources for, 102–104
    technology and, 98–102
    see also knowledge
liabilities, 80–81
lifelong learning, 95–96
lifestyle, 9–10
life-work balance, 37
LinkedIn, 67, 102–103
lists, shopping, 79
longevity, 186, 188, 190
    see also aging
Longevity Paradox: How to Die Young at a Ripe Old Age (Gundry), 179
Lowenstein, Roger, *Buffett: The Making of an American Capitalist*, 86
Lyubomirsky, Sonja, *How of Happiness, The*, 142

Index

MacDonald, Mrs. Ramsay, 60
Mandela, Nelson, 15
Massachusetts Male Aging Study, 157
mastermind group, 53–54
materialism, 135
math skills, 41
McGill, Bryant H., 114
McKeever, Teri, 134
meal planning, 77, 80
   see also dietary guidelines; foods
medications, 162
mediocrity, 21–23
meditating, 129–130, 145–146, 160, 174–175
MedlinePlus, 176
Melinda, Gates, 85
memory, 153–154, 157–161
memory rescue, 154–156
mental state, 56
mercury, 162
Michael Breus, *Power of When, The*, 56
mindset, 30–32
mission statements, 15–16
money
   aging and, 67–69
   happiness and, 87–88
   management of, 63–67, 79–87, 89–91
   saving, 69–75
   spending habits and, 65–67, 77–87

spending wisely, 75–76, 147
morality, 134
Morrill, Sam, "New Couple Gets Quarantined," 110
Morrison, Toni, 14
motivations, 12–13, 35–37

nature, 184
needs, essential, 43
negative advice, 22–23
negativity, 20–21, 45–46, 173–174
neglectfulness, 25
networking, 40
"New Couple Gets Quarantined" (Morrill and Tomlinson), 110

obsessions, 22
occipital lobes, 157
one-cent option, 24
online instruction, 101
opportunities. see SWOT (strengths, weaknesses, opportunities, threats)
optimism, 132
oral care, 179
overspending, 75–76
owning vs renting, 91

Panafric Hotel (Kenya), 57
PANAS (Positive Affect and Negative Affect Schedule), 150
parietal lobes, 156

passions, 33
PCBs (polychlorinated biphenyls), 162
peace of mind, 11
Peale, Norman Vincent, *Art of Living, The*, 60
perfectionism, 171–172
persistence, 54–55
personal fulfillment, 104–105
personal growth, 11
personalities, toxic, 20
pesticides, 163, 164
physical activities, 176–178
Pinterest, 80
plan, action, 26–27
plaques, 158
pollutants, air, 163
polychlorinated biphenyls (PCBs), 162
positivity
    achievements and, 57
    aging and, 187–190
    causes of, 143–145
    emotional contagion and, 20–21
    gratitude and, 125–127
    happiness and, 139, 141, 145–148
    humor and, 110–113
    vs negativity, 13
    practicing, 136–137
posture, 58
Power of When, The (Breus), 56

praying, 129, 160
prefrontal cortex, 156
priorities, 12, 60
problem-oriented approach, 21
productivity, 56, 113
public speaking, 39
purchases, planning for, 72–74

quality, 81
questions, asking, 59
questions, for self-reflection, 28–30

Rand, Ayn, 142
reality, current, 10–11
reinventing yourself, 12
relationships, 11, 60–62, 132, 186–187
relaxation, 41
relief theory, 108
renovating, 81
renting vs owning, 91
repairing vs replacing, 72
repetition, 46–47
researching, 41, 59, 74
responsibilities, 18–19, 38
retirement, working after, 67–69
roadblocks to spending, 82
Rockefeller, John D., Sr., 61
rumination, 173–174

Index

sacrifices, 37–38
safety, 110
salt, 180
Satisfaction with Life Scale (SWLS), 150
saving money, 81
Schultz, Howard, 57
Science of Getting Rich, The (Wattles), 130
Second City, The, 109
self-control, 132–133
self-esteem, 20–21, 174
selfishness, 87
self-management, 40
Senior Net, 103
sex, 185–186
shopping, comparison, 74
shopping lists, 79
SHS (Subjective Happiness Scale), 150–151
signature strength, 148
Silver Surf, 103–104
Skype, 101
sleep, 135, 161
smiling, 114–116
smoke, 163
social media, 190
Social Security, 105
solidarity, 110
solution-oriented approach, 21

spending, 65–67, 77–87
Squawk Box, 84
standards of excellence, 25–27
Start Late, Finish Rich (Bach), 70
strengths, 33
   see also SWOT (strengths, weaknesses, opportunities, threats)
stress management, 175–176
strokes, 159
Subjective Happiness Scale (SHS), 150–151
substitutions, 75
success
   aging and, 190–193
   commitment for, 47–51
   compounding development effect and, 23–25
   defining, 9–10
   goals and, 42–47
   gratitude and, 130–131, 136
   growth mindset for, 30–32
   happiness and, 37, 140–141
   humor and, 109–113
   joyful living and, 60–62
   mastermind groups and, 53–54
   mental state and, 56
   never too late for, 14–15
   persistence and, 54–55
   positivity and, 51–53
   sacrifices for, 37–39
   seeking, 12–13, 190–193

Index

   skills for, 39–42
   strategies for, 35–37
sunshine, 184
superiority theory, 108–109
supplements, 161
sweeteners, artificial, 163
SWLS (Satisfaction with Life Scale), 150
SWOT (strengths, weaknesses, opportunities, threats), 26

TAN (Third Age Network), 93–94
tech savviness, 98–101
TechBoomers.com, 101
technological advances, 98–101
Technology for Seniors Made Easy, 104
telomere, 173
temporal lobes, 156
Think and Grow Rich (Hill), 53
Third Age Network (TAN), 93–94
threats. *see* SWOT (strengths, weaknesses, opportunities, threats)
tidiness, 58–59
Tomlinson, Taylor, "New Couple Gets Quarantined," 110
Toronto Metropolitan University, 94
toxic personalities, 20
toxins, 161–167
traveling, 80, 184–185
Trello (app), 104
triggers, 11–12
Twain, Mark, 108

Underground Value (blog), 86

values, 32–33
Veenhoven, Ruut, 149
vitamins, 161, 180–181, 184
volunteering, 102, 187

walking, 177
Wattles, Wallace, *Science of Getting Rich, The*, 130
weaknesses. *see* SWOT (strengths, weaknesses, opportunities, threats)
wealth, 65–67
　see also financial security
well-being, 131, 143
Wilde, Oscar, "Work is the curse of the drinking classes," 109
wine, red, 180
"Work is the curse of the drinking classes" (Wilde), 109
working after retirement, 67–69
working smarter, 56–58
workplace, humor and, 110–113
workshops, 102
World Database of Happiness, 149
World Happiness Day, 149
writing, 39–40

YouTube videos, 101

Zussman, Shirley, 185

About the Author

M.M. Amon is a member of The Institute of Sales & Marketing Management of the United Kingdom. A graduate of Long Island University, Amon has worked as a radio broadcaster and journalist in Rwanda, and a sales executive in the hospitality industry in Kenya.

Originally from Rwanda, Amon currently makes his home in London, Ontario. *How to Succeed After 55* is his first book.

www.ingramcontent.com/pod-product-compliance
Lightning Source LLC
Chambersburg PA
CBHW031106080526
44587CB00011B/851